NUTRITION AND DIET RESEARCH PROGRESS

COMPREHENSIVE GUIDE TO NUTRITION IN POLYCYSTIC OVARIAN SYNDROME (PCOS)

NUTRITION AND DIET
RESEARCH PROGRESS

Additional books and eBooks in this series can be found on Nova's website under the Series tab.

NUTRITION AND DIET RESEARCH PROGRESS

COMPREHENSIVE GUIDE TO NUTRITION IN POLYCYSTIC OVARIAN SYNDROME (PCOS)

ANNCHEN WEIDEMANN

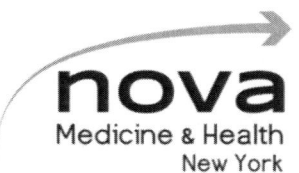

nova
Medicine & Health
New York

Copyright © 2019 by Nova Science Publishers, Inc.

All rights reserved. No part of this book may be reproduced, stored in a retrieval system or transmitted in any form or by any means: electronic, electrostatic, magnetic, tape, mechanical photocopying, recording or otherwise without the written permission of the Publisher.

We have partnered with Copyright Clearance Center to make it easy for you to obtain permissions to reuse content from this publication. Simply navigate to this publication's page on Nova's website and locate the "Get Permission" button below the title description. This button is linked directly to the title's permission page on copyright.com. Alternatively, you can visit copyright.com and search by title, ISBN, or ISSN.

For further questions about using the service on copyright.com, please contact:
Copyright Clearance Center
Phone: +1-(978) 750-8400   Fax: +1-(978) 750-4470   E-mail: info@copyright.com

NOTICE TO THE READER

The Publisher has taken reasonable care in the preparation of this book, but makes no expressed or implied warranty of any kind and assumes no responsibility for any errors or omissions. No liability is assumed for incidental or consequential damages in connection with or arising out of information contained in this book. The Publisher shall not be liable for any special, consequential, or exemplary damages resulting, in whole or in part, from the readers' use of, or reliance upon, this material. Any parts of this book based on government reports are so indicated and copyright is claimed for those parts to the extent applicable to compilations of such works.

Independent verification should be sought for any data, advice or recommendations contained in this book. In addition, no responsibility is assumed by the Publisher for any injury and/or damage to persons or property arising from any methods, products, instructions, ideas or otherwise contained in this publication.

This publication is designed to provide accurate and authoritative information with regard to the subject matter covered herein. It is sold with the clear understanding that the Publisher is not engaged in rendering legal or any other professional services. If legal or any other expert assistance is required, the services of a competent person should be sought. FROM A DECLARATION OF PARTICIPANTS JOINTLY ADOPTED BY A COMMITTEE OF THE AMERICAN BAR ASSOCIATION AND A COMMITTEE OF PUBLISHERS.

Additional color graphics may be available in the e-book version of this book.

Library of Congress Cataloging-in-Publication Data

ISBN: 978-1-53615-655-3
Library of Congress Control Number: 2019942947

Published by Nova Science Publishers, Inc. † New York

To all women suffering with the condition of PCOS, and in particular those who are desperate to fall pregnant.

To my two daughters, Dr. Jana Groenewald and Dr. Anneke Weidemann for their continued support and motivation.

CONTENTS

List of Tables		ix
List of Figures		xi
Preface		xiii
Acknowledgments		xv
List of Acronyms and Abbreviations		xvii
Part I	**The Science behind the Disorder of Polycystic Ovary Syndrome (PCOS)**	1
Chapter 1	About Polycystic Ovarian Syndrome	3
Chapter 2	Factors in the Pathophysiology of PCOS	27
Chapter 3	Brief Overview of Drugs and Surgery Used for Treatment in PCOS	81
Chapter 4	Alternative and Complementary Treatments for Use in PCOS	87
Chapter 5	PCOS in Adolescence	101

Part II	**Nutritional Considerations and Treatment Strategies for the Woman with PCOS**	**109**
Chapter 6	The Optimal Diet for PCOS	**111**
Chapter 7	New Dietary Strategies for Treatment in PCOS	**137**
References		**147**
Author's Contact Information		**163**
Index		**165**
Related Nova Publications		**169**

LIST OF TABLES

Table 1.	Criteria for identifying the metabolic syndrome in women with PCOS	**34**
Table 2.	Examples of foods containing high and low AGEs	**51**
Table 3.	Carbohydrate composition (%) of commercial sweeteners	**61**
Table 4.	Sugar content of selected common fruit and vegetables (g/100g)	**63**
Table 5.	Names and examples of aromatic amines	**72**
Table 6.	Foods rich in folate/folic acid	**96**
Table 7.	Trans-fat contents of food	**121**
Table 8.	Good sources of non-heme iron compared to some best sources of heme iron	**126**

LIST OF FIGURES

Figure 1. The stages of development of the ovarian follicle — **9**

Figure 2. The carefully controlled ebb and flow of hormones in the normal menstrual cycle — **12**

Figure 3. Hormonal interactions during the early follicular phase. — **14**

Figure 4. The structure of the ovarian follicle — **14**

Figure 5. The cysts around the periphery of the ovaries seen on transvaginal ultrasound, referred to as the "string of pearls" — **17**

Figure 6. The hormonal imbalance through hyperinsulinemia at the core of PCOS — **31**

Figure 7. The steps in the Maillard reaction — **48**

Figure 8. The AGE-RAGE interaction — **50**

Figure 9. Different hepatic pathways of fructose and glucose. — **58**

Figure 10. The putative mechanisms that link fructose excess to MS — **65**

Figure 11. Ovarian follicle: 85 days of development — **113**

Figure 12. The mean insulin scores for 1000kJ (240 calorie) portions of 38 different foods — **123**

PREFACE

Polycystic ovarian syndrome (PCOS) is the single largest cause of infertility in women of childbearing age, with the incidence having risen from around 15% to 21% within 6 – 8 years. Not only has the incidence risen in this population, but in adolescents, PCOS is being diagnosed earlier and more frequently than ever before.

There is no written "diet" or single food that cures PCOS, but factors from Westernized eating such as trans fats, advanced glycation end-products and fructose overload are factors which affect both the development of PCOS and the resistance to drug-related treatment of it. For the woman with PCOS, whether trying to fall pregnant of manage symptoms, it is of cardinal importance to understand that a "diet mentality" is inappropriate, since the entire lifestyle should be changed to favour the menstrual cycle and the production of its hormones for at least three months prior to expecting normal ovulation. The awakening and development of the primordial follicle destined to become the ovulatory one, 85 days prior to ovulation, points to the compulsory consistency of improved eating habits and lifestyle. Almost every single food/meal/drink/snack has an influence on your ovulatory capacity. It is imperative that the PCOS woman seeking help for either symptomatic relief or fertility, understands the relationship of the hormonal chaos of PCOS to the hormonal chaos of a poor diet.

The standard dietary composition of 20% protein, 50% carbohydrate and 30% fat was used to treat PCOS since the beginning of research, after the discovery of PCOS as Stein-Leventhal syndrome in 1935. Weight loss was known to be the most important factor in treating PCOS, but no progress was made, and the drop-out rate of diets given to these women was extremely high. For some reason, women with PCOS could not adhere to a formal diet, and battled weight loss, although small studies could not confirm this. The answer to this probably lies in the disturbance of their hunger and satiety cascade, regulated by insulin.

New drugs have seen the light and were tested on females with PCOS with mediocre results, showing that something else but the PCOS was at play.

This book is dedicated to show the power and strength of poor dietary habits (and visa versa) on drug treatment of PCOS, and the lack of need for it when dietary habits and lifestyles are improved. In PCOS, drugs could probably never win over a poor eating lifestyle, which is a point often missed by fertility specialists eager to help with a quick fix, rather than a longer process that can be maintained over the long-term.

The mere fact that in women undergoing IVF treatment, end-stage-glycation products were found in their oocytes, tells a story of the horrendous effect of poor dietary habits on fertility.

Both the keto-genic diet and intermittent fasting (done under professional dietetic supervision), either apart or together, have provided a means for quicker and safer weight loss, especially if time is of the essence in older couples.

ACKNOWLEDGMENTS

1. Mariette Nortje, for her thorough editing and language care of this document.
2. Nova Science Publications who offered me the opportunity to create this book from more than 15 years of work and study in the field of PCOS, although in a private capacity.

LIST OF ACRONYMS AND ABBREVIATIONS

AA	arachidonic acid
AE-PCOS	Androgen Excess and PCOS (Society)
AGEs	advanced glycation end-products
AI	artificial insemination
ALA	alpha linolenic acid
AMH	anti-Müllerian hormone
ApoB	apolipoprotein B100
ART	assisted reproductive technology
ASRM	American Society for Reproductive Medicine
BED	binge-eating disorder
BI	bioelectrical impedance
BMI	body mass index
CC	clomiphene citrate
CCK	cholecystokinin
CLA	conjugated linoleic acid
CNS	central nervous system
CoA	co-enzyme A
COH	controlled ovarian hyper stimulation
CR	caloric restriction
CRP	C-reactive protein
CT	computed tomography

CVD	cardiovascular disease
DCI	D-chiro-inositol
DFE	dietary folate equivalent
DHA	docosahexanoic acid
DHEA	Dehydroepiandrosterone, also known as androstenolone
DHEA-S	Dehydroepiandrosterone sulfate, also known as androstenolone sulfate
DNA	deoxyribonucleic acid
DNL	de novo lipogenesis (converting excess carbohydrates into lipids for storage, by the liver. Lipid is much more energy-dense than carbohydrate and is therefore a more efficient storage form).
EPA	Eicosapentanoic acid
ESHRE	European Society for Human Reproduction and Embryology
Estradiol (E2)	mainly produced by the ovaries for follicle growth and maturation
Estriol (E3)	mainly produced during pregnancy
Estrone (E1)	mainly the variant of estrogen produced in fat cells, to serve as a reservoir of estrogen, as the female body ages
FDA	US Food and Drug Administration
FFA	free fatty acids
FSH	follicle stimulating hormone
GI	glycemic index
GL	glycemic load
GLUT4	glucose transporter type-4
GLUT5	glucose transporter type-5
GnRH	gonadotropin-releasing hormone
GRAS	generally regarded as safe
H	Androgen excess
HbA1c	haemoglobin A1c
HDL	high-density lipoprotein (cholesterol)
HFCS	high-fructose corn syrup

List of Acronyms and Abbreviations

HIV	human immunodeficiency virus
HOMA-IR	homeostatic model assessment of insulin resistance
HPO-axis	hypothalamic-pituitary-ovarian-axis
HRQoL	health-related quality of health
IGF-1	insulin-like growth factor 1
IGT	impaired glucose tolerance
IL-1β	interleukin-1 beta
IL-6	interleukin-6
IPGs	inositolphosphoglycans
IR	insulin resistance
IVF	in vitro fertilization
LDL	low-density lipoprotein (cholesterol)
LEPR	leptin receptor
LH	luteinizing hormone
MI	Myo-inositol
MS	metabolic syndrome
MTHFR	methylenetetrahydrofolate
NAC	N-acetyl-cysteine
NAFLD	non-alcoholic fatty liver disease
NAS	National Academy of Sciences (of the USA)
NASH	non-alcoholic steatohepatitis
NF-κB	nuclear factor kappa-B
NHS	Nurses' Health Study
NICE	National Institute of Clinical Excellence
NIH	National Institutes of Health (of the USA)
NSAID'a	non-steroidal anti-inflammatory drugs
O	oligo/anovulation
OCPs	oral contraceptive pills
OGTT	oral glucose tolerance test
OHSS	ovarian hyperstimulation syndrome
P	polycystic ovarian morphology
PCOS	polycystic ovarian syndrome
PFK	phosphofructokinase
POF	premature ovarian failure

PPARs	peroxisome proliferator-activated receptors
PUFA	poly-unsaturated fatty acid
QoL	quality of life
RAGE	the cell receptor for AGEs
RCOG	Royal College of Obstetricians and Gynaecologists
RCT	randomized controlled trial
REE	resting energy expenditure
RNA	ribonucleic acid
ROS	reactive oxygen species
SHBG	sex hormone-binding globulin
SIRT-1	silent information regulator-1
SOGC	Society of Obstetricians and Gynecologists of Canada
sRAGE	soluble RAGE
SREBP	sterol receptor-binding protein
TCD	total caloric deprivation
T2DM	type-2 diabetes mellitus
TNF-α	tumour necrosis factor alpha
TZD	troglitazone
USA	United States of America
VLDL	very-low-density lipoprotein
WC	waistline circumference
WHR	waist-hip-ratio

Part I:
The Science behind the Disorder of Polycystic Ovary Syndrome (PCOS)

Chapter 1

ABOUT POLYCYSTIC OVARIAN SYNDROME

1.1. HISTORY OF POLYCYSTIC OVARIAN SYNDROME

In 1935, two gynaecologists from Chicago, Irving Stein and Michael Leventhal described an unusual cluster of symptoms in seven of their patients: excess facial and body hair, irregular menstrual periods and enlarged ovaries filled with cysts. The condition was initially known as Stein-Leventhal syndrome, but today we refer to it as polycystic ovarian syndrome or PCOS. (Chavarro, Willett & Skerrett, 2008; Roe & Dokras, 2011).

Because of PCOS, the ovulatory function of the ovaries is affected. Therefore, many women are diagnosed after they realise that pregnancy is not forthcoming, despite their efforts. Initially considered as an infertility problem, PCOS is now recognised as a metabolic condition, with serious long-term health consequences (Agapova et al., 2014; Herriot, Whitcroft & Jeanes, 2008; Macut et al., 2017; Marsh & Brand-Miller, 2005; Rotterdam, 2003).

Throughout literature, various names have been used to describe the same disorder (Szydlarskam, Machaj & Jakimiuk, 2017):

- Functional ovary androgenism;
- Hyperandrogenic, chronic anovulation;
- Ovarian dysmetabolic syndrome;
- Polycystic ovarian syndrome;
- Polycystic ovaries disorder;
- Polycystic ovary syndrome;
- Sclerotic polycystic ovary syndrome;
- Syndrome of polycystic ovaries.

Although generally regarded as such, Stein and Leventhal were not the first investigators into PCOS. In 1721, an Italian medical scientist, physician, and naturalist, Vallisneri, described: "Young married peasant women, moderately obese and infertile, with two larger than normal ovaries, bumpy, shiny and whitish, just like pigeon eggs". In 1884 Chereau, and in 1855, Rotikansky, described fibrous and sclerotic lesions on the ovaries of a degenerative character, containing fluid-filled follicles (Kar, 2013, Szydlarska et al., 2017).

In 1879, Lawson Tait published in the British Medical Journal about the need for bilateral removal of ovaries (oophorectomy), which were of degenerative, cystic nature, causing symptoms. After partial resection of the ovaries was proposed, Von Kahlden published a review in 1902 in Germany, on the pathology and clinical implications of such degenerative ovaries. Ovarian resection was heavily criticized, and in 1915, John A. McGlinn suggested surgically puncturing "those cysts which are upon the surface" instead of resorting to removal of the ovaries (Szydlarska et al., 2017).

Stein and Leventhal suggested surgical intervention ("wedge resection") in order to reduce the size of the ovary, and avoid removing the entire ovary. All seven of the cases in their investigation resumed normal menstrual cycles after this surgery, and two fell pregnant. With development of less invasive medical treatment for ovarian stimulation, surgical intervention is performed infrequently (Szydlarska et al., 2017).

Hippocrates (460-377 BC) referred to the influence of obesity on menstruation. In his essay about "the influence of climate, water supply and health situation," he referred to women with impaired reproductive function as follows: "...the girls become flaccid and pudgy... persons with this constitution cannot generate many children... fat and flaccidity are the culprits. The uterus is unable to receive semen and the women menstruate little and in an infrequent manner" (Rodriguez et al., 2009). Hippocrates further noted: "But those women whose menstruation is less than three days or is meagre, are robust, with a healthy complexion and a masculine appearance; yet they are not concerned about bearing children nor do they become pregnant".

Moises Maimonides (1135-1204 AD), a medieval physician noted: "There are women whose skin is dry and hard, and whose nature resembles the nature of a man. However, if any woman's nature tends to transform to the nature of a man, this does not arise from medications, but is caused by heavy menstrual activity." The famous French surgeon and obstetrician, Ambroise Paré (1510-1590 AD) observed: "Many women, when their flowers of tearmes be stopped, degenerate after a manner into a certain manly nature, whence they are called Viragines, that is to say stout, or manly women; therefor their voice is loud and bigge like unto a man's, and they become bearded" (Azziz, Dumesic & Goodarzi, 2011).

In 2011, Azziz et al., published an article entitled *Polycystic ovary syndrome: An ancient disorder?* The authors embarked on trying to answer their title question, in the light of PCOS having had evolutionary/survival advantage, and therefore persisted, in spite of its reproductive disadvantage.

It is possible that PCOS had its origins in Paleolithic hunter-gatherer communities? The males, females and offspring with the greatest capacity for energy storage, would endure and survive prolonged periods of deprivation and other environmental stressors. This genotype (the set of genes in our deoxyribonucleic acid or DNA) is often referred to as the "thrifty gene". As a result, the body becomes "thrifty" with energy loss. The resting energy expenditure (REE), as well as the heat produced after eating a meal (postprandial thermogenesis), are diminished in this genotype. The reduction in energy expenditure would necessarily mean that the body becomes more able to improve energy stores, probably mainly as fat, but also as lean body mass (Azziz et al., 2011).

Among nomadic hunters, it would have been advantageous and maybe necessary for women to space their children, as they could only carry and care sufficiently for one child at a time. In antiquity (and present-day Africa), mortality from childbirth-related complications was high, and a lower parity may have served to reduce the death rate of women in reproductive age, and the risk of abandonment of the offspring. Another advantage would have been better food availability and protection to fewer children, and because of their inherited genotype, these children would have been better able to survive periodic deprivation. Another interesting argument is that females with PCOS may have supported the survival of the family unit. Women with few or no children could have served as child-minders, to those who had to hunt and gather, and with increased muscle, fat stores and bone density, these women may have created a reliable source of child-rearing labour, not threatened by pregnancy (Azziz et al., 2011).

The authors concluded that it is indeed plausible that the PCOS genotype could have been transmitted over several generations by children conceived between fertile carrier males and sub-fertile carrier females. The improved energy utilization and greater sturdiness of affected women could have contributed to their reduced capacity to conceive children, which served both to reduce maternal mortality, and prove a rearing advantage for their children and kin (Azziz et al., 2011).

1.2. The Female Reproductive System

1.2.1. An Introduction to Follicles

Every healthy female is born with all the follicles (or immature egg-cells) that she could utilize during her natural life, packed into both ovaries. Of the approximately two million eggs a female is born, around eleven thousand die every month, prior to puberty. From the age of puberty, a woman has 300 000 to 400 000 remaining eggs, and from this point, 1 000 eggs are destined to die monthly. This inexorable death of egg cells is independent of hormone production, birth control, nutritional supplementation, lifestyle, pregnancies or ovarian stimulation or inhibition by artificial means. When the ovarian supply of eggs ceases, the production of estrogen by the ovaries is stopped, and the woman goes into menopause. There is no such similar phenomenon in men, despite the journalistic hype. During their lifetime, men continue to produce testosterone and sperm at virtually the same rate, with only a very modest decline as they age (Silber, 2018).

To have a better understanding of how an ultrasound examination can help find one's place on one's biological clock, bear in mind that roughly 35 eggs die every day (amounting to the 1 000 per month). Each of these eggs had started their emergence from a resting pool of eggs, on a long, three-month journey of development towards becoming an egg, capable of ovulation. Every month only one egg (out of the 1 000 follicles that started the process) will make it to the fullest maturity, ovulating a mature, fertilizable egg into the fallopian tubes. This quiet "awakening" process of the daily 35 eggs is signaled by some process still not fully understood by science, and the three-month development process is totally dissociated from the menstrual or ovulatory cycle. Only once the three-month-stage of the awakened follicles reaches the antral stage (see Figure 1), they finally become sensitive and susceptible to the hormones of the monthly menstrual cycle (Silber, 2018).

1.2.2. The First Eighty-Five (85) Days of Follicle Development

Most of the 300 000 to 400 000 follicles in the female ovaries, are inert during any given month, except for the average of 35 that begin awakening for development each day. During the first 70 days of development, the follicle is completely independent of any menstrual hormonal influence or hormonal events that have taken place in previous cycles. After 70 days, these follicles, now known as antral follicles, will have grown to a size of about two millimetres (2mm), at which time they are visible with high-quality ultrasound scanning. They are now sensitive to the influence of follicle stimulating hormone (FSH) from the pituitary gland (Silber, 2018).

The number of follicles leaving the "resting pool" is inversely related to the age of the woman, and her declining fertility. In a 20-year old woman, an average of 35 follicles will leave the resting pool daily, whereas, in a 35-year old woman, an average of 10 follicles per day leave the resting pool.

The reader is encouraged to understand the normal mechanisms involved in the maturation of the ovarian follicle to the desired end-point, ovulation, in order to understand the imbalance that causes the condition of PCOS to develop. This way, the mechanisms for causing failure to ovulate, or produce a mature egg of good quality would be better understood, and the dietary guidelines in the second part of this book will make better sense.

1.2.3. The Normal Development of Ovarian Follicles during the Menstrual Cycle

Follicular development does not start and end during the menstrual cycle, but rather starts before birth, in the uterus, during development of the ovaries in the fetus. At birth and during childhood, the ovaries contain only primordial follicles, and hormonal stimulation for starting growth and maturation begins during puberty. Some follicles may remain in the primordial stage for up to 50 years, before "waking up" and going through the stages of development. The time lapse between the primordial stage to a mature follicle ready for ovulation, could be 6 to 12 months. Through the stages of development, many follicles stop and die, and only one percent (1%) of all follicles will ever develop to a mature oocyte (egg), for ovulation. (Gurevich & Sadatay, 2018).

All the follicles in the ovary start as very small primordial follicles, impossible to see via ultrasound. Every day, from the onset of puberty, hormonal influences cause some of the primordial follicles to start "awakening" and maturing. Should the follicles survive, they graduate through stages of growth. In the tertiary stage the follicle forms a fluid-filled cavity, known as the antrum (see Figure 1) and the follicles are known as antral follicles. The antral follicles are almost 200 times larger than a primordial follicle, and typically measure two to ten millimetres (2-10mm).

They are now visible on ultrasound examination, usually done transvaginally (Gurevich & Sadatay, 2018).

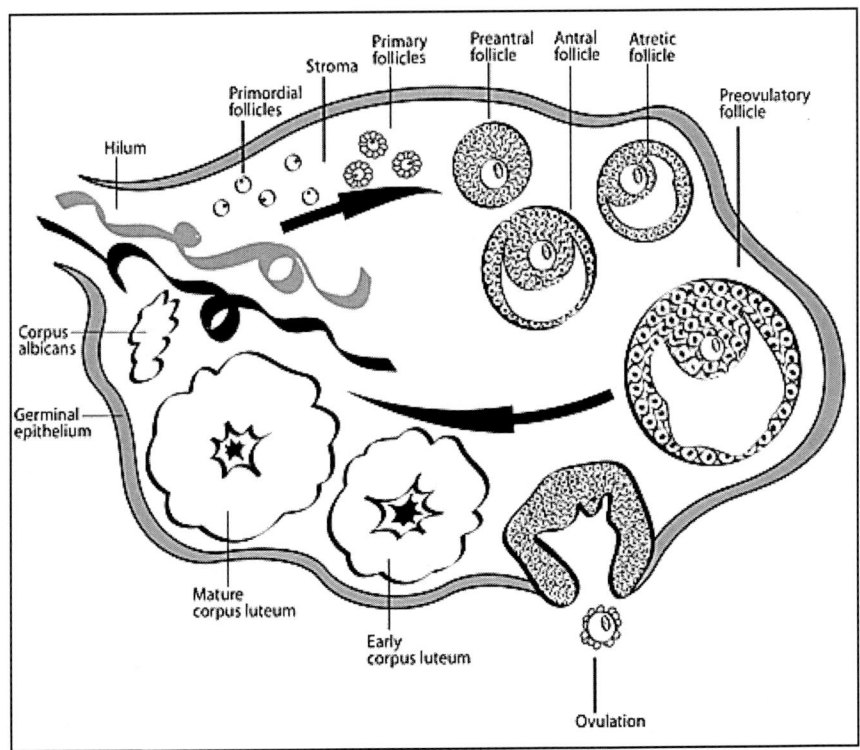

Source: Silber, 2018.

Figure 1. The stages of development of the ovarian follicle.

In theory, if it were possible to know the number of follicles inside the ovaries, one would have a good idea of the number of potential eggs present, or in the case of older women, the number of follicles left for potential development. Unfortunately, it is impossible to count the number of follicles, as they are too small to visualise until they have developed into antral follicles. The number of active antral follicles on the ovary correlates to the number of follicles left. Although there still is no way to know the exact number of follicles, a woman with very few antral follicles developing, probably has a low ovarian reserve of follicles (Gurevich & Sadatay, 2018). Although several follicles are stimulated from each ovary, to begin maturing during a menstrual cycle, normally only one will undergo ovulation from either ovary, or set free a mature egg. Almost 99% of ovarian follicles will disintegrate and never reach maturity to release an egg.

1.3. STAGES OF FOLLICLE DEVELOPMENT

As illustrated in Figure 1, the female reproductive cycle is split into two phases: (1) the follicular phase preceding ovulation; and (2) the luteal phase. In the follicular phase, follicles in the tertiary stage of development are stimulated and recruited to begin the process that will eventually lead to ovulation. The primary responsibilities of the follicles are to protect the developing oocyte, releasing reproductive and stimulatory hormones. After ovulation, the follicles comprise the corpus luteum which means "yellow body" in Latin, and from which the hormone progesterone is released (Chavarro, 2008; Gurevich & Sadatay, 2018).

The following sequence of events takes place in a predictable manner every four weeks in females during the reproductive years and is described in several publications:

1. *Primordial follicle*: These follicles are at the resting stage.
2. *Primary follicle*: From puberty until menopause, an average of 35 primordial follicles are activated daily to start developing. The oocyte enlarges, and granulosa cells start dividing to form layers. A primary follicle contains two layers of granulosa.
3. *Secondary follicles*: More than two layers of granulosa cells surround the oocyte. Theca cells (see Figures 1 and 4) start developing, after five layers of granulosa cells, giving structure to the follicle and starting hormonal secretion.
4. *Tertiary follicles*: The follicles now contain a fluid-filled cavity and are known as antral follicles. They are visible with transvaginal ultrasound examination, and they are now sensitive to the hormonal changes of the monthly menstrual cycle (Gurevich & Sadatay, 2018; Silber, 2018).

5. *Mature follicle*: The follicle is now fully mature, awaiting the surge of hormones to break open and release the oocyte into the fallopian tubes during ovulation for possible fertilization (Gurevich & Sadatay, 2018; Silber, 2018; Young & McNeilly, 2010).
6. *Corpus luteum*: Technically this is no longer a follicle, although it appears on the surface of the ovary for a short while. It constitutes the open follicle that released the mature oocyte (Gurevich & Sadatay, 2018; Silber, 2018).

1.3.1. The Hormonal Cascade in Follicle Development

Hormones play a complex role in fertility and the journey from the follicle to the fertilized egg (ovum). Several hormones are involved in the monthly cycle of ovulation and the preparation for a possible pregnancy.

Hormones are signaling molecules produced in the endocrine glands, and they are circulated through the body by means of the circulatory system. Hormones regulate the functioning and behaviour of distant organs. There are two types of hormones: (1) peptide hormones and (2) steroid hormones.

Peptide hormones are water-soluble and perform their actions through binding to the surface of target cells via cell receptors, signaling the desired outcome through one or more messengers over the cell membrane. In this book, peptide hormones are discussed under Section 2.12: "The role of appetite regulation in PCOS".

Steroid hormones are made from the structure of the molecule cholesterol, and are fat-soluble. They move through both the outer and the nuclear membranes of their target cells and act in the nucleus of the cell. Steroid hormones are mainly the sex hormones (estrogen, androgens, and progesterone). Not only the gonads (sex organs: testicles, ovaries and uterus) are able to produce steroid hormones, but the adrenal glands and fat cells can also produce smaller amounts of steroid hormones such as estrogen and testosterone (Funder et al., 1997).

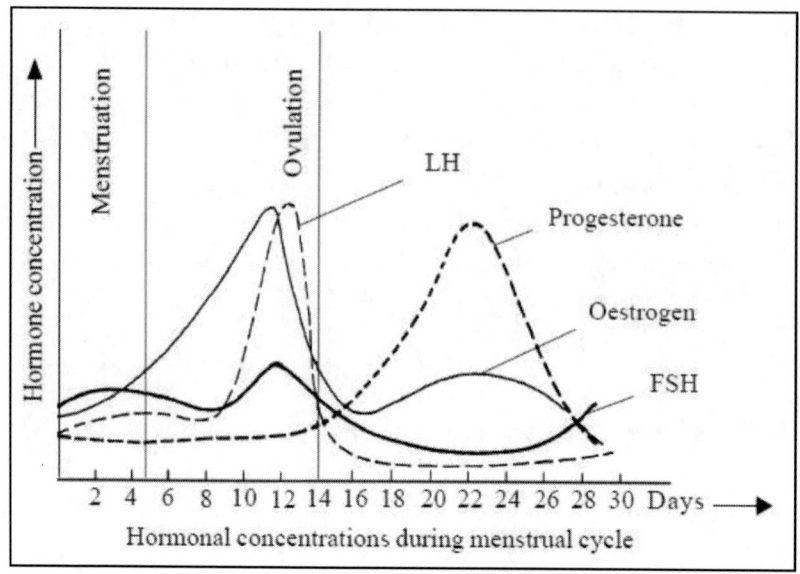

Source: Othman, 2010.

Figure 2. The carefully controlled ebb and flow of hormones in the normal menstrual cycle.

The hormones involved in the growth and maturation of follicles on the ovary during each menstrual cycle are:

- Gonadotropin-releasing hormone (GnRH);
- Follicle stimulating hormone (FSH);
- Luteinizing hormone (LH);
- Estrogen (steroid hormone):
  - Estrone (E1) (mainly the variant of estrogen produced in fat cells, to serve as a reservoir of estrogen, as the female body ages)
  - Estradiol (E2) (mainly produced by the ovaries for follicle growth and maturation)
  - Estriol (E3) (mainly produced during pregnancy)
- Progesterone (steroid hormone):
  - Androstenedione (mainly produced and functions in the ovaries)

- Dehydroepiandrosterone (DHEA), also known as androstenolone and dehydroepiandrosterone sulphate (DHEA-S) (mainly produced by the adrenal glands)
- Testosterone (produced equally by the adrenal glands and the ovaries).

In the brain, the hypothalamus, situated directly behind the eyes, sends out pulses of GnRH. This in turn stimulates the pituitary gland (in a different part of the brain) to release FSH and LH into the bloodstream. FSH serves to provoke a cluster of follicles in each ovary to begin maturing, mainly by multiplying the granulosa cells of the follicle, which will produce estrogen under the influence of FSH. LH mainly contributes to the process by stimulating the theca cells to produce androgens and other substances, which are precursors of estrogen.

Estrogen has several roles to fulfil in the menstrual cycle. As the levels of estrogen rise, produced by the influence of FSH on maturing follicles, feedback to the pituitary gland results in decreased production of FSH and LH, slowing the growth of all but the most matured follicle. The slowed follicles that do not reach the stage of ovulation, undergo disintegration, a process known as atresia. A surge in LH and FSH serves as the trigger for ovulation (Chavarro et al., 2008; Gurevich & Sadatay, 2018).

LH is responsible for converting the eggless remains of the ovulation into the corpus luteum (see Figure 1). In response to LH, the corpus luteum produces progesterone. Progesterone is necessary to prepare and stabilize the endometrium for implantation of a possible pregnancy, and stimulates the development of new blood vessels (Chavarro et al., 2008).

The synchronized actions of the hormones, starting with GnRH from the hypothalamus, through FSH and LH secretion by the pituitary gland, is also known as the hypothalamic-pituitary-ovarian-axis (HPO-axis) (Chavarro et al., 2008; Grassi, 2013; Roe & Dokras, 2011).

During the maturation process, LH mainly stimulates the actions of the theca cells, while FSH stimulates the actions of the granulosa cells (see Figures 3 and 4) (Guet et al., 1999; Magoffin, 2005).

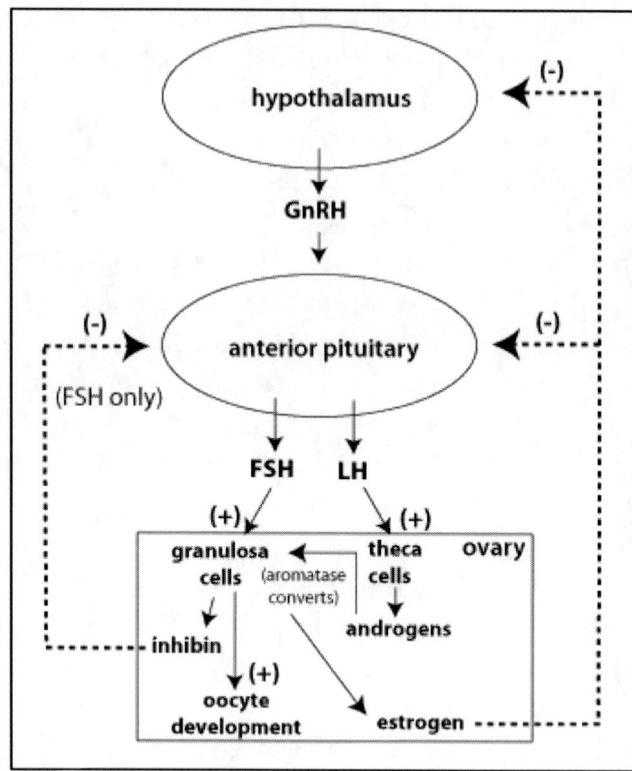

Source: University of Washington, 2018.

Figure 3. Hormonal interactions during the early follicular phase.

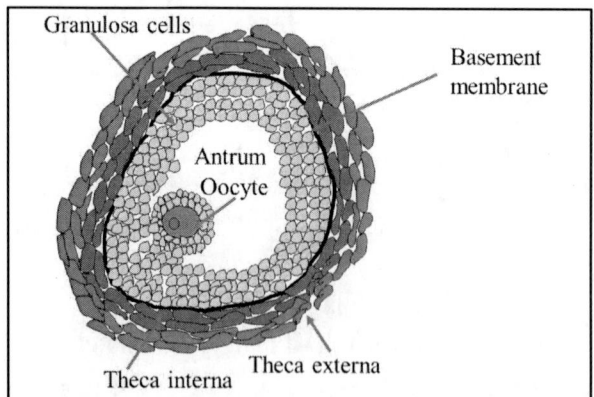

Source: Wilson, 2019, slide 9.

Figure 4. The structure of the ovarian follicle.

1.3.2. Importance of Theca and Granulosa Cells

Theca cells are exclusively found in the ovary and specifically as part of the maturing follicle. Providing both structure and support, the theca cells are vital components of the developing follicle.

Theca cells are also the exclusive producer of ovarian androgens (mostly androstenedione), which are necessary as substrates for estradiol and estrone production in the nearby granulosa cells.

After activation, follicles are thought to recruit precursor theca cells from surrounding ovarian tissue (ovarian stromal tissue) around the granulosa cells and oocyte. Theca cells, granulosa cells and the oocyte form the follicle structure that produces steroid hormones. Steroid hormones are manufactured from cholesterol as the backbone of these hormones. The functions of theca cells include not only producing androgens, but also providing crucial signals to the granulosa cells and oocyte during follicular development (Young and McNeilly, 2010).

Androgens are produced through a desmolase enzyme in the theca cells, and are transferred to the granulosa cells, where an FSH-stimulated enzyme, known as aromatase, converts the androgens into estrone and estradiol (the estrogen variants that stimulate the dominant oocyte to mature, and signal the pituitary gland to decrease FSH and stimulate LH). Over-activity of the theca cells could also stimulate the fat cells of the body, which contain aromatase, to produce estrone. This means that peripheral to the ovary, estrogen can be produced in fat cells and also give feedback to the hypothalamus regarding the regulation to release FSH and LH. Either hyperactivity or hypoactivity of the theca cells can lead to infertility. Hyperactivity leads to hyperandrogenism or androgen excess, while hypoactivity leads to lack of estrogen, mostly in the form of estradiol, from the ovary.

Insulin plays an important role in theca cell function, and studies have been shown to induce dose-dependent cell multiplication, and increased steroid production, through increased expression of certain related genes (Magoffin, 2005; Young & McNeilly 2010). Research from 1997 supports the hypothesis that PCOS is characterized by an intrinsic abnormality of theca cell androgen production (Gilling-Smith et al., 1997).

Both theca and granulosa cells play a vital role in the pathogenesis of PCOS, and the reader is encouraged to take note of these two cell-types in developing follicles, in order to better understand the mechanisms that might cause PCOS, also known as the pathophysiology, or the origins of how the syndrome might develop.

1.4. The Impact of PCOS on the Menstrual Cycle

A carefully controlled cascade of hormones stimulates a few follicles on each ovary to start maturing during a menstrual cycle. Once matured, ovulation occurs to set the mature follicle free on its path through the fallopian tubes, to encounter sperm for fertilization. The ovum is implanted into the endometrium, resulting in pregnancy. In the woman with PCOS, the hormonal cascade has gone awry through one or more of several factors (see Figure 4), and the maturing follicles remain trapped in the ovary instead of being released at ovulation. The follicles do not develop into maturity, which is also known as "follicular arrest".

The acronym PCOS refers to *poly* (many) *cystic* (cysts or fluid-filled sacs, which are actually follicles) *ovarian* (on the ovary) *syndrome* (including a set of associated conditions).

The unreleased follicles seen in the syndrome of PCOS become multiple small cysts throughout the ovary, causing the capsule around the ovary to swell and the ovary to increase in size (Chavarro et al., 2008). The classic picture on a transvaginal ultrasound of the ovary presents the picture of a "string of pearls," which describes the appearance of cysts on at least one ovary (see Figure 5). The multiple cysts are normally situated around the periphery (outer surface) of at least one ovary (Grassi, 2013; Lucidi, 2018).

About Polycystic Ovarian Syndrome 17

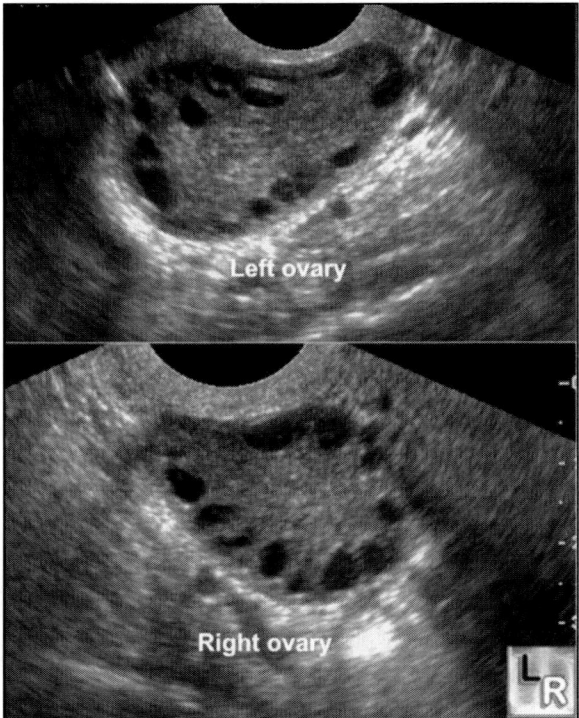

Source: Learning radiology, 2018.

Figure 5. The cysts around the periphery of the ovaries seen on transvaginal ultrasound, referred to as the "string of pearls".

In 2011, Azziz and colleagues performed a study of more than 300 women with PCOS. The women treated with placebo ovulated at around one-third of the expected ovulation frequency, implying that women with PCOS are able to conceive, but at a rate lower than normal. Women with PCOS are not infertile, but sub-fertile. (Azziz et al., 2011).

1.5. CLINICAL PRESENTATION OF PCOS

1.5.1. Measurable, Clinical Symptoms

The American Society of Reproductive Medicine Practice defines 'infertility' as a condition of "failure to conceive after twelve of more moths of attempts of natural fertilization", and is estimated to affect 50 to 80 million women in their reproductive age, or up to 50% of women worldwide in this category (Silvestris et al., 2018).

The syndrome of PCOS is accompanied by one or more of the following symptoms (Chavarro et al., 2008; Grassi, 2013; Lucidi, 2018; Macut et al., 2017):

- Amenorrhea (no menstrual period) or oligomenorrhea (menstrual irregularity);
- Anovulation with resulting infertility;
- Hyperandrogenism (elevated blood levels of male hormones):
  - Hirsutism (unwanted hair growth, mostly facial hair but also other body parts)
  - Alopecia (loss of scalp hair, or male-like balding)
  - Acne (facial area and on the back)
- Polycystic ovaries on sonographic examination;
- Obstructive sleep apnea;
- Insulin resistance (IR):
  - Acanthosis nigricans (darkening of the skin, especially around the neck) and skin tags around the neck and under-arm areas
  - Abdominal fat accumulation (with or without overweight/obesity)
  - Overweight or obesity
  - Hypertension
- Psychological symptoms such as depression and low self-esteem.

Aptly but sadly, PCOS is also referred to in literature as "the thief of womanhood" (Sikaris, 2004). PCOS sufferers are prone to depression, low self-esteem, and shame about their outward symptoms, such as hair growth, acne, weight gain and abdominal fat. They often have a sense of failure because they cannot seem to control these symptoms with their best efforts. The devastating realisation that they may have difficulty or might be unable to bear children adds to the psychological distress of the woman with PCOS (Grassi, 2013).

1.5.2. Subjective, Self-Reported Symptoms

Apart from these clinical symptoms, which can be measured in some way, there are also an array of subjective clinical symptoms mostly self-reported by undiagnosed sufferers of PCOS, and sadly not recognised by many practitioners, because of their subjective nature.

In 2008, Herriott et al. did a retrospective audit of 88 patients who had been treated for PCOS at a private clinic during the course of two years. Both lean and overweight PCOS patients attended the clinic, and data from both their medical and dietetic records was available. The number of lean PCOS patients was almost double that of overweight PCOS patients (58 and 30 respectively).

The study reported that 17% of patients had a previous or current form of eating disorder, which is a statistic higher than that reported for the general population by research elsewhere. In 1991 and 1995, data had been published observing the association between PCOS and bulimia (Herriott et al., 2008).

Fifty-nine patients (70%) in the study reported cravings for carbohydrates, and the cravings were equally distributed between lean and overweight PCOS subjects. Lean PCOS patients reported symptoms of hypoglycaemia (described as 'shaky', 'light-headed', or 'dizzy') more frequently than overweight PCOS patients (73% and 43% respectively). Abdominal weight gain was reported by 93% of overweight patients, as opposed to 47% of lean PCOS patients, and hunger was also more frequently reported (86%) by overweight patients, than by lean patients (43%) (Herriott et al., 2008).

It should be noted that, amongst the group of lean PCOS patients, abdominal weight gain and hunger were reported by almost half of the patients. A feeling of lethargy and tiredness was reported by 82% of all the patients in the study. Gastro-intestinal symptoms, described as irritable bowel syndrome (constipation and uncomfortable bloating), or a perceived intolerance to certain foods, were reported by 67% of all patients, irrespective of lean or overweight status. More patients were vegetarian or semi-vegetarian (16%) than statistics reported for the general population (Herriott et al., 2008).

Quality of life (QoL) plays a large role in the life of a PCOS sufferer, with the condition already having been labelled "the thief of womanhood", as has been noted earlier. The symptomatic presentation of the patient, together with frustration regarding the weight gain and the loss of previous feminine characteristics, form an important whole in the treatment of PCOS. The inability to produce children further exacerbates the condition, with the patient coming to rely on empathy and support from the clinician, whatever the discipline might be.

1.5.3. Depression, Anxiety, Quality of Life, and Disordered Eating

The abnormalities of reproductive and metabolic features in females with PCOS have been well described, but few studies have investigated the emotional well-being, mood-disorders and health-related quality of health (HRQoL) in this subgroup of females. The economic and health burden due to the high prevalence of PCOS (12% to 21%) amongst women of child-bearing age, mandates the understanding of this condition across the board of its clinical features, including psychological well-being (Dokras et al., 2018).

Women with PCOS commonly report symptoms of depression, such as fatigue, sleep disturbance and general lack of interest (Dokras et al., 2018). Some researchers have cited obesity as the primary cause of reduced HRQoL in PCOS, and many have reported frustration with the seeming inability to lose weight, giving rise to poor body image and low self-esteem. In a meta-analysis by Dorkas et al. (2018), it was confirmed that the depressive symptoms were independent of BMI. Two other studies in the meta-analyses reported increased clinical diagnoses in women with PCOS, and in Australia, the incidence of depression in women with PCOS was significantly higher in women with PCOS as opposed to non-PCOS women.

Therefore, the need for screening PCOS females for symptoms of depression is becoming pressing. In the future, the screening for depression should also explore the different PCOS phenotypes (Dokras et al., 2018).

Females with PCOS also seem to experience increased symptoms of anxiety, and anxiety disorders. A study of 16 weeks of physical exercise, did not find a difference in anxiety scores, and the subjects did not lose weight. There is some evidence that a high protein, low carbohydrate diet for 16 weeks improved depression scores as opposed to a low protein, high carbohydrate diet, although there was no difference in weight loss between the two groups (Dokras et al., 2018).

Hirsutism seems to be a distressing factor for females with PCOS. A study from Iran showed hirsutism as having the greatest overall impact on HRQoL (Dokras et al., 2018). Thomson et al., (2010) cited a study where improved psychological health was observed, after six months of laser treatment for facial hirsutism.

In the study by Thomson et al., 2010, three PCOS groups of females were compared for HRQoL after a 20-week intervention with diet only (14 subjects), diet and aerobic exercise (15 subjects) and diet combined with aerobic-resistance exercise (20 subjects). The study showed that diet in overweight and obese PCOS women improved depression and HRQoL scores, but the addition of exercise provided no additional benefit to diet alone.

The prevalence for disordered eating in women with PCOS ranges from 12% to 36%. Although in the general population, there is a clear association between binge-eating disorder (BED) and obesity, data on the PCOS population is very limited and the impact of PCOS-related treatment on disordered eating is unclear. Research in the fields of HRQoL, depression and anxiety, and disordered eating is sorely needed to broaden the holistic approach to PCOS and offer appropriate treatment after screening results (Dokras et al., 2018).

1.6. Definition and Diagnosis of PCOS

Since the original description in 1935, the definition of PCOS has undergone several revisions (Chavarro et al. 2008; Roe & Dokras, 2011). No single diagnostic criterion can be used, and PCOS diagnosis should exclude disorders which mimic the PCOS phenotype (the physical expression of the trait) (Rotterdam, 2003). Three distinct sets of diagnostic criteria have been developed for diagnosis of PCOS in adult females (Agapova et al. 2014; Grassi, 2013; Lucidi, 2018; NIH, 2012; Roe & Dokras, 2011). The outcomes of these diagnostic criteria are discussed below.

1.6.1. NIH 1990 Criteria

The United States National Institutes of Health (NIH), sponsored an expert conference in 1990, around suitable criteria for the diagnosis of PCOS. The following two diagnostic criteria for PCOS were proposed:

1. Chronic anovulation (or oligo-ovulation manifested by menstrual irregularity) (Lucidi, 2018; Rotterdam, 2003); and
2. Evidence of clinical or biochemical hyperandrogenism (evidence of androgen excess).

Other disorders resulting in menstrual irregularity and hyperandrogenism, which could mimic the PCOS phenotype (e.g. congenital adrenal hyperplasia, androgen-secreting tumours, or Cushing syndrome) should be excluded (Lucidi, 2018).

1.6.2. Rotterdam 2003 Criteria

In 2003, the Rotterdam European Society for Human Reproduction and Embryology (ESHRE) and the American Society for Reproductive

Medicine (ASRM) sponsored a consensus workshop group, and proposed that the diagnosis include two of the following three criteria:

1. Oligo- and/or anovulation;
2. Clinical and/or biochemical hyperandrogenism;
3. Polycystic ovaries demonstrated on transvaginal ultrasound.

Other etiologies which mimic PCOS must be excluded, as with the 1990 NIH criteria, including hyperprolactemia, and a severe form of acanthosis nigricans, HAIRAN syndrome, and high dose exogenous androgens (Lucidi, 2018; Roe & Dokras, 2011; Rotterdam, 2003).

1.6.3. AE-PCOS Criteria of 2006 & 2009

The Androgen Excess and PCOS (AE-PCOS) Society, led by Azziz et al., published a position statement (2006) and a task force report (2009) (Azziz et al., 2009). They emphasized that PCOS is primarily a disorder of androgen excess, and its diagnosis should thus include all three of the Rotterdam criteria with hyperandrogenism (hirsutism/hyperandrogenemia) as a definitive criterion:

1. Clinical hyperandrogenism (hirsutism) of biochemical hyperandrogenism (elevated total/free testosterone);
2. Ovarian dysfunction (oligo-menorrhea or oligo-ovulation);
3. Polycystic ovaries on transvaginal ultrasound examination.

All three criteria are necessary to fulfil the diagnosis of PCOS, after exclusion of other causes of androgen excess (Lucidi, 2018; NIH, 2012; Roe & Dokras, 2011).

1.6.4. NIH 2012 Criteria

The final report of the 2012 NIH workshop recommended using the Rotterdam criteria (which includes the NIH and AE-PCOS criteria), and also specifying the phenotype in all research studies and clinical care (Kar, 2013; Makut et al., 2017; Penaforte et al., 2009).

The four phenotypes are:

1. Androgen excess + oligo/anovulation (H + O);
2. Androgen excess + polycystic ovarian morphology (H + P);
3. Oligo/anovulation + polycystic ovarian morphology (O + P);
4. Androgen excess + polycystic ovarian morphology + oligo/anovulation (H + P + O) (also referred to as "PCO complete" or "classic PCOS").

There is little research into the significance of the phenotypes with regard to metabolic and long-term complications. However, a 2013 study, which was the first to investigate the phenotypes in a large cohort of women, shed some light. The most prevalent phenotype seemed to be the "PCO complete" or "classic PCOS" (H + P + O), and the least prevalent, the ovulatory phenotype, i.e. androgen excess + PCO morphology (H + P). This seems to be the case in similar studies in other countries, such as Turkey, Bulgaria and Iran. The phenotype that does not show androgen excess (O + P) is referred to as a "mild" form of PCOS (Kar, 2013).

Females with classic PCOS are more prone to abdominal obesity, displaying more prevalent dyslipidemia, insulin resistance (IR) and metabolic syndrome. These women also show more pronounced hyperandrogenemia than other phenotypes.

Even the mild form of PCOS (O + P) shows prevalent metabolic syndrome, and in the absence of hyperandrogenemia, develops IR in the presence of obesity. Still unknown, is how the different phenotypes of PCOS evolve with aging (Makut et al., 2017).

Due to the intrinsic characteristics and the highly heterogenous nature of the symptoms, the diagnosis of PCOS has not been fully standardised, and is still being questioned and debated in recent literature. The classical form of PCOS seems to pose a strong independent risk for impaired glucose tolerance and type-2 diabetes mellitus (T2DM). Furthermore, classic PCOS includes most or all of the symptoms of metabolic syndrome, such as abdominal fat accumulation and insulin resistance, hence posing a greater risk for developing cardiovascular disease (CVD) (Penaforte et al., 2009).

1.7. PREVALENCE AND HEALTH RISKS OF PCOS

The incidence of PCOS has risen to epidemic proportions, since its first description in medical literature in 1935 with an incidence of less than one percent (1%) (Arora, 2017). It is now recognized that PCOS is the most common endocrine disorder in all women of reproductive age (Herriot et al., 2008; Marsh & Brand-Miller, 2005; Roe & Dokras, 2011). PCOS represents the cause of 75% of cases of anovulatory infertility in the population of women of reproductive age (Moran et al., 2013; Rencber et al., 2018).

PCOS is a heterogenous condition, involving females of all ethnicities, in all countries of the world. The syndrome affects an estimated 6% to 25% of females in their reproductive years, with a higher prevalence in South Asian countries, reported at 50% (Arora, 2017). This suggests a thorough and clear understanding of the underlying causative factors for PCOS. Insight into the metabolic and hormonal disturbances is essential to address women's health and expand knowledge on ways to treat this multi-faceted syndrome (Macut et al., 2017).

Dyslipidemia, or a deranged cholesterol profile, is the most prevalent metabolic aberration in PCOS. The lipid-profile is most frequently one typical of atherogenic dyslipidemia, including hypertriglyceridemia, low levels of high-density lipoprotein (HDL) cholesterol and increased levels of small, dense low-density lipoprotein (LDL) cholesterol. This places women with PCOS at increased risk for cardiovascular and cerebrovascular disease (Grassi, 2013; Lucidi, 2018; Macut et al., 2017; Teede, Hutchinson & Zoungas, 2007). Hyperandrogenism is independently linked to increased risk of cardiovascular disease (CVD) in PCOS (Macut et al., 2017).

PCOS is also associated with a high risk for impaired glucose tolerance (IGT) and type-2 diabetes mellitus (T2DM). (Lucidi 2018; Saleem & Rizvi, 2017). Whether the incidence of CVD in PCOS is increased over non-PCOS females remains unclear, but both the conditions of IGT and T2DM are significant factors in the development of CVD (Teede et al., 2007).

Both lean and obese PCOS women should be screened for diabetes before the age of 30, and those who test negative, should have ongoing screening throughout their lifetime (Lucidi, 2018). The increased risk for T2DM and gestational diabetes, could be the cause for spontaneous abortion or miscarriage. In women with PCOS, the rate of early pregnancy loss is 30% to 50%, which is three-fold higher than in non-PCOS women. It is reported that 36% to 83% of females who suffer early loss of pregnancy have PCOS. Recent literature reports that hyperinsulinemia adversely affects the endometrial environment and functions, which could lead to implantation disturbance and/or early pregnancy loss (Sakumoto et al., 2010).

PCOS also increases the risk for endometrial hyperplasia and carcinoma, since chronic anovulation causes constant stimulation of the endometrium with estrogen, without progesterone. Suitable induction of withdrawal bleeding should be done with progestogens every 3 to 4 months. As the Royal College of Obstetricians and Gynaecologists (RCOG) reported no known association with ovarian or breast cancer, no additional screening is needed (Ludici, 2018).

Women with PCOS also show an increased incidence of obstructive sleep apnea, which is regarded as an independent risk factor for CVD. Questioning the patient on daytime somnolence might be a starting point for referral for a sleep assessment (Lucidi, 2018).

Non-alcoholic fatty liver disease (NAFLD) represents the accumulation of excessive fat in the liver, and obesity and insulin resistance seem to be key factors in its development.

Chapter 2

FACTORS IN THE PATHOPHYSIOLOGY OF PCOS

2.1. OVERVIEW

Despite enthusiastic scientific interest and research into PCOS through the past decade, there is still controversy over many of its facets, such as diagnosis, prevalence, pathogenesis, long-term risks, drug treatment, and especially the dietary and lifestyle management of the condition. The clinical and biochemical features of PCOS may vary according to ethnicity. Furthermore, criteria used for diagnosis, and the features of PCOS may change during the lifetime of the woman (Kar, 2013; Moran & Norman, 2004).

Most studies and opinions in research literature agree that insulin resistance (IR) and high circulating levels of insulin, underpin the development of the syndrome in both lean and overweight females, and IR is implicated in disruption of the HPO-axis, causing ovulatory dysfunction. However, several of these studies include comments that the exact cause of PCOS is yet unknown (Kar, 2013; Marsh & Brand-Miller, 2005; Moran & Norman, 2004). Recently, genetic factors and embryonic exposure to high levels of androgens from the mother have received increasing attention as a possible cause for PCOS (Arora, 2017; Klein, 2018; Macut et al., 2017).

The symptoms of PCOS are mainly caused by the following two factors:

- Hyperinsulinemia/insulin resistance (IR); and
- Hyperandrogenemia.

Since these conditions mostly co-exist in PCOS (with the exclusion of one phenotype), there has been debate on which of the two hormonal excess conditions existed first, and which one causes the other. There is good evidence that high levels of insulin are the primary contributing factor to production of excess androgens in the ovaries (Arora, 2017):

- Pharmocological interventions to lower insulin levels in PCOS, result in reduced levels of androgens;
- When both ovaries are surgically removed to alleviate androgen excess in PCOS, it has no effect on hyperinsulinemia or on insulin resistance.

Most researchers agree that insulin resistance is a key metabolic defect in the development of PCOS (Arora, 2017; Moran & Norman, 2004, Teede et al., 2007). However, not all women with PCOS will exhibit IR or hyperinsulinemia. The measurement of IR has been controversial for many years, but the most accurate measures are largely inaccessible and used mainly for research purposes. Other methods, such as the homeostatic model assessment of insulin resistance (HOMA-IR) value, which gives the proportionate value between fasting insulin and fasting glucose could be used to measure insulin resistance (Huang, 2009).

2.2. THE EFFECT OF INSULIN ON PCOS

There is a difference between hyperinsulinemia and insulin resistance (IR), which is important for the reader to understand. Not all females with high levels of circulating insulin are insulin resistant. Insulin resistance must combine with dysfunction of the β-cells (the cells on the pancreas that secrete insulin) or failure of these cells to secrete sufficient insulin, and hence show impairment in glucose clearance (glucose intolerance). Only when the effectivity of the insulin starts to show inability to regulate blood glucose the diagnosis of IR is justified (Teede et al., 2007; Weidemann & Brand, 2016).

The hormone insulin is produced by the beta-cells (β-cells) of the pancreas, and stimulated mainly by dietary intake when the blood sugar levels rise above a carefully-controlled level. The sugar absorbed from food is of no use to the body cells while circulating in the blood, as it cannot flow freely into the cells without help. Glucose must pass through a molecular "gate" on the cell membrane, which only insulin can open. Upon the "unlocking" action of insulin on the cell, glucose transporter type-4 (GLUT4) multiply rapidly at the surface of the cell, facilitating the influx of glucose into the particular cell. The GLUT4 is insulin-dependent in most tissues. Once inside the cell, glucose is phosphorylated by the enzyme glucokinase, and the intracellular metabolism of glucose begins (Chavarro et al., 2008; Weidemann, 2012).

The definition of insulin resistance is the inability of insulin to exert its biological effect, being glucose clearance from the blood and directing it into body cells for use or storage. This results in a feedback mechanism to the β-cells of the pancreas, mainly on stimulation from dietary intake, to secrete more insulin, resulting in high levels of circulating insulin, with adverse metabolic effects (Sakumoto et al., 2010). As the pancreas continues to over-produce insulin, the β-cells become more dysfunctional, to the detriment of the effectivity and sufficiency of insulin. Elevation of insulin levels probably far precedes (by as much as a decade) the actual rise in glucose, which follows the failure of the β-cells of the pancreas, after prolonged over-stimulation through compensatory hyperinsulinemia. Furthermore, it is well known that compensatory hyperinsulinemia and insulin resistance are triggered by obesity, and more specifically, the cells of accumulated visceral or abdominal fat (Sakumoto et al., 2010). The liver also decreases in its ability to remove insulin from the bloodstream (Moran & Norman, 2004).

Comprehensive reviews exist on insulin resistance in PCOS, and current understanding supports the existence of *intrinsic or unique IR* in PCOS (Gambineri et al., 2012), which is mechanistically different from the *extrinsic IR* (Moran et al., 2013) related to obesity, adverse dietary intake and the use of anabolic steroids (Arora, 2017). The intrinsic IR in PCOS is directly related to the β-cell dysfunction as described above, by which β cells show impaired biological response to both endogenous (produced by the body) and exogenous (injected into the body) insulin, giving rise to disturbed metabolic and cell productive processes (Teede et al., 2018).

Intrinsic IR is also present in lean females with PCOS, as shown by Stepto et al. (2013). Twenty (20) overweight and twenty (20) lean PCOS subjects were taken off insulin sensitizers for 3 months, and compared in an academic setting to 14 overweight and 19 lean non-PCOS controls. The subjects were tested using the hyperinsulinemic-euglycemic clamp technique in an academic setting. This method of testing for insulin resistance is not suitable for the public at large, and usually only done in controlled research settings. The plasma insulin concentration is raised and maintained at a known level, while glucose is infused at variable rate, until a "steady-state" is reached. The glucose infusion rate now equals the glucose uptake by all the tissues in the body, and is regarded as the measure of tissue insulin sensitivity (Von Wartburg, 2007). In the Stepto study, 75% of the lean PCOS women were insulin resistant, and 95% of the overweight PCOS women were insulin resistant. To illustrate the exacerbating effect of obesity, 62% of the non-PCOS, overweight controls, were found to be insulin resistant (Stepto et al., 2013).

2.3. Effect of Insulin on the HPO-Axis

Through disturbance of the carefully-controlled cascade of hormones released during the menstrual cycle by the HPO-axis, insulin causes increased pulsality of GnRH by the hypothalamus, priming the pituitary gland to favour an increase of LH over FSH. The ratio of LH to FSH now reverses and LH becomes dominant over FSH (ratio > 2).

With insufficient levels of FSH, the granulosa cells and oocytes of the maturing follicles stop growing, and FSH is unable to stimulate the enzyme aromatase to produce estrogen (estradiol) from aromatizable androgens. The feedback mechanism from estradiol on the pituitary gland becomes insufficient to balance the levels of FSH and LH, and LH production escalates (see Figure 6).

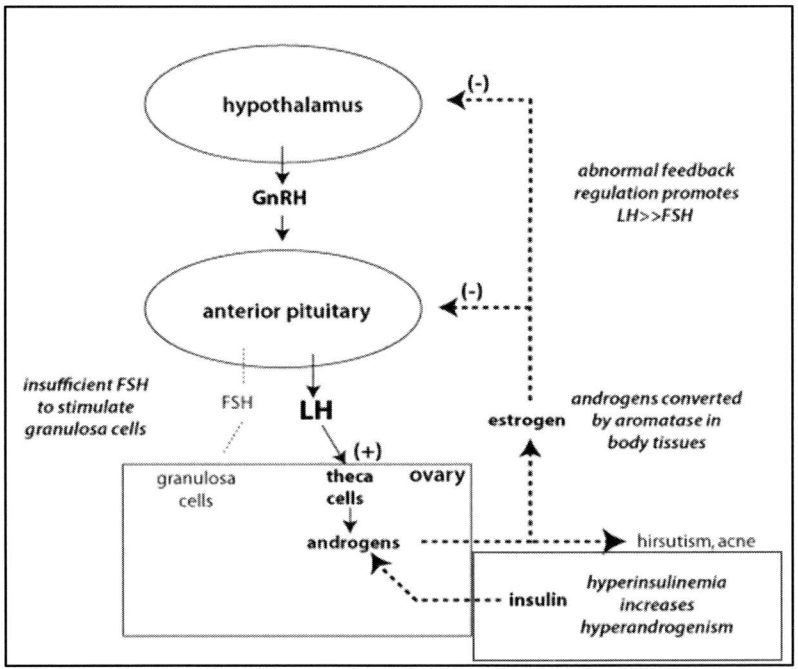

Source: University of Washington, 2018.

Figure 6. The hormonal imbalance through hyperinsulinemia at the core of PCOS.

The incidence of PCOS is more frequently observed in females with both type-1 and type-2 diabetes, regardless of body composition. This observation might imply the causative effect of endogenous (internally produced) or exogenous hyperinsulinemia on increased ovarian production of androgens (Macut et al., 2017).

Hyperinsulinemia is also known to cause a condition called acanthosis nigricans for which the Latin meaning is "black skin." Darker discolouring of the skin is especially noticeable in people with darker skin-tone, and is easily detected around the entire neck area (sometimes more so on the back of the neck), elbows, knees, knuckles, underarms, between the breasts and across the groin. The more severe the insulin resistance, the more pronounced the acanthosis nigricans. Another feature of hyperinsulinemia may be skin tags, which appear as loose keratin follicles around the neck and other areas of the body, or reddened inflamed or rough hair follicles on the upper arms (Grassi, 2013).

Hyperinsulinemia may also stimulate receptors for insulin-like growth factor-1 (IGF-1). This hormone is a potent growth hormone, with positive effects on growth in childhood, but questionable effects in adults with elevated levels. IGF-1 stimulates the androgen production by LH further. This leads to suppression of the production of the binding hormone for IGF-1 by the liver. At the same time, insulin suppresses the production of another binding hormone, sex hormone-binding globulin (SHBG) by the liver, contributing to the increase in free androgen levels (Arora, 2017; Sakumoto et al., 2010). The situation of high insulin, excess androgens and high levels of IGF-1, causes clinical symptoms of androgen excess (Arora, 2017).

Many factors, such as lifestyle, disease, body mass index (BMI) and eating habits, could affect the production of SHBG. Low levels of SHBG do not necessarily only correlate with high androgen levels, but rather with the presence of IR/high circulating insulin levels. (Sakumoto et al., 2010; Teede et al., 2007; Weidemann, 2012).

2.4. Insulin Resistance, PCOS and the Metabolic Syndrome

Insulin resistance and hyperinsulinemia are also known causes for the development of metabolic syndrome (MS), which is characterized by impaired glucose tolerance (IGT) or type-2 diabetes mellitus (T2DM), hypertension, abdominal obesity and increased risk for CVD (Arora, 2017; Moran & Norman, 2004; Penaforte et al., 2009).

Women with PCOS show an 11-fold higher risk of MS, a set of risk factors that increase the risk for diabetes and CVD. It is reported that 35% to 40% of adults with PCOS have MS (Agapova et al., 2014; Kar, 2013). The PCOS population with the highest occurrence of MS is reported in India, with a prevalence of 46.2%. Obese PCOS women had a three- to four-fold higher prevalence of MS compared to lean PCOS women. Abnormal waistline circumference (WC) and reduced levels of HDL-cholesterol were the major components of MS that were presented by lean PCOS women. Therefore, it is recommended that lean patients with PCOS also be regularly screened for MS (Kar, 2013).

Abdominal/visceral obesity and insulin resistance, act synergistically with the development of reproductive and endocrine abnormalities that characterize PCOS. Insulin resistance is known to be a major contributor to or metabolic susceptibility factor in the development of MS (Essah & Nestler, 2006; Farshchi et al., 2007; Kandaraki, Christakou & Diamanti-Kandarakis, 2009). Evidence shows that the presence of MS increases the risk of atherosclerotic vascular disease two-fold, and the onset of T2DM five-fold. PCOS has similarly been associated with an increased risk for both CVD and diabetes, and most of the symptoms of MS are also prevalent in PCOS. The suggestion has been made that PCOS might be a gender-specific form of MS. Additional metabolic components might not specifically form part of the formal definitions of MS, but include the presence of a pro-thrombotic state, increased inflammatory markers, elevated uric acid levels, obstructive sleep apnoea, and non-alcoholic steatohepatitis (NASH) (Essah & Nestler, 2006).

The Rotterdam (2003) consensus group and other consensus conferences have advised against the screening for insulin resistance, because of concerns regarding the value of these tests. In the place of this, criteria have been developed to define the metabolic syndrome, a condition that includes components associated with and underpinned by insulin resistance, as explained above. These components include abdominal or visceral obesity, hypertension, elevated fasting glucose and dyslipidemia.

The Rotterdam consensus group advised that obese women with PCOS should be screened for metabolic syndrome and for glucose intolerance through an oral glucose tolerance test, evaluating the fasting glucose and 2-hour glucose level after a 75g glucose challenge for intolerance (Rotterdam, 2003).

Table 1. Criteria for identifying the metabolic syndrome in women with PCOS

	Risk factors	Cut-off levels
1.	Abdominal obesity measured as waist circumference	> 88 cm (35 in)
2.	Triglycerides	>1.70 mmol/l (> 150 mg/dl)
3.	HDL-cholesterol	< 1.2 mmol/l (< 50 mg/dl)
4.	Blood pressure	>130/>85 mmHg
5.	Oral glucose tolerance test:	
	Fasting	3.5 to 5.5 mmol/l
	2 hours glucose	> 7.8 mmol/l

Of the four phenotypes of PCOS (see Section 1.6: "Definition and diagnosis of PCOS"), the hyperandrogenic phenotypes presented with a four- to five-fold higher prevalence of MS (37% to 50%), compared with the non-hyperandrogenic phenotype (O + P), with a prevalence of 10% (Kar, 2013).

2.5. INSULIN RESISTANCE, HYPERANDROGENISM AND PCOS

There are consistent reports in literature that hyperinsulinemia correlates positively with hyperandrogenemia in both lean and overweight PCOS women, when compared to weight-matched controls (Moran & Norman, 2004). Hyperandrogenism is connected with the inflammatory profile and oxidative stress that accompanies the clinical profile of PCOS (Gonzalez, 2015; Rencber et al., 2018; Sakumoto et al., 2010). The importance of regarding the relationship between obesity (hyperinsulinemia/IR) and excessive androgen production is as follows (Pasquali, 2006):

- Obesity exerts a profound influence on sex-hormone production and metabolism;
- Androgens play a pinnacle role in regulating the distribution of body fat according to sex;
- Changes in levels of androgens may create favourable grounds for endocrine disorders, such as PCOS;
- Sex-hormone imbalance is bound to cause infertility in both males and females;
- Androgen excess is known to favour the development of co-morbidities, such as T2DM and CVD.

In general, sex hormones do not travel freely through the bloodstream, but are accompanied by a "chaperone." This ensures that the sex hormones do not exert their effect for too long and/or on inappropriate tissues. As mentioned, the chaperone, sex hormone-binding globulin (SHBG) is manufactured by the liver and has a larger affinity for testosterone than for estrogen (Chavarro et al., 2008). In the face of hyperandrogenism resulting from increased theca cell production of androgens from over-secretion of LH, production of SHBG by the liver is reduced, giving rise to elevated free androgens, especially testosterone (Sakumoto et al., 2010).

Non-PCOS women presenting with significant insulin resistance could have regular menses and normal levels of androgens. It has also been found that, in the majority of hyperandrogenemic women with PCOS, the excess androgen production is predominantly ovarian, and not adrenal. This might indicate that PCOS women tend to harbour an intrinsic theca cell defect, leading to ovarian hyper-production of androgens, independently of extra-ovarian factors (Gilling-Smith et al., 1997; Kandaraki et al., 2009).

2.6. Obesity and Fat Distribution

The World Health Organization has set standards and cut-off points for the classification of underweight, normal weight, overweight and obesity for adults above 18 years of age. The measurements are based on body mass index (BMI), which comprises (weight in kg) ÷ (length in metres)^2. The unit of BMI is set mass in kg/(height in m)^2 and comprises the body surface area (Weidemann & Brand, 2016):

- < 18.5 kg/m^2 = underweight;
- 19 to 25 kg/m^2 = normal weight;
- >25 to 30 kg/m^2 = overweight;
- >30 kg/m^2 = obesity.

The BMI has several shortcomings, in that it does not distinguish between male and female, body frame size, and body fat mass as opposed to lean body muscle (muscle weighs more than fat). The extremes on the BMI scale (underweight due to intentional 'dieting' or starvation (BMI < 19 kg/m^2) and obesity due to poor quality hyper-nutrition, show negative outcomes in terms of fertility. Extreme thinness and extreme obesity affect the ovarian function and are associated with decreased pregnancy rates, and higher miscarriage events. High BMI in both PCOS and non-PCOS women is associated with adverse pregnancy outcomes such as gestational diabetes, hypertension, and premature delivery (Silvestris et al., 2018).

It is estimated that six percent (6%) of all women are morbidly obese (BMI > 35 kg/m^2), and the negative effects of obesity on the reproductive function of women is well known: As opposed to normal-weight women, obese women frequently undergo menstrual irregularity and disorders of ovulation, endometrial pathology, and infertility. Overweight and obesity also cause impairment in assisted conception programs. Furthermore, due to poor oocyte quality, obesity is often associated with negative outcomes for patients undergoing in vitro fertilization (IVF).

Obesity and PCOS share several common features in their development. In order to attain better understanding of which condition comes first, more research is needed (Saleem & Rizvi, 2017). Within the population of PCOS females, the incidence of obesity is reported as ranging between 38% and 88%. The history of weight gain usually precedes the onset of oligomenorrhea and hyperandrogenism, which suggests a pathogenic role of obesity in the development of PCOS. The causes for the prevalence of obesity in PCOS have been unclear, but genetic factors as well as environmental factors have been shown to play key roles (Penaforte et al., 2009). The accumulation of abdominal fat might confer increased health risks, with evidence that abdominal/visceral fat correlates more strongly with metabolic syndrome, than subcutaneous fat. Abdominal obesity is more common in females with PCOS than same-weight women without PCOS, and worsen the clinical features of infertility, correlating strongly with increased androgens and LH levels (Moran & Norman, 2004).

Excessive abdominal adiposity characterizes all weight classes of PCOS – normal weight, overweight and obese (González, 2015). Abdominal obesity in PCOS contributes towards insulin resistance, probably through subclinical inflammation (Macut et al., 2017). Obesity in PCOS is also associated with endothelial dysfunction and other markers of systemic inflammation (except for adiponectin, which seems to protect against inflammation), exacerbating the development of CVD (Farshchi et al., 2007; Marsh & Brand-Miller, 2005).

Elevated levels of C-reactive protein (CRP) have been shown in women with PCOS (Marsh & Brand-Miller, 2005), together with inflammatory cytokines such as tumour necrosis factor-alpha (TNF-α), interleukin-6 (IL-6), iterleukin-18 (IL-18) and a host of other markers of systemic inflammation (Rencber et al., 2018). The cytokines, which mainly bring about inflammatory response, are hormone-like compounds, mainly released by visceral fat, increasing the risk of CVD (Farshchi et al., 2007). Weight loss in overweight or obese patients would have the additional benefit of reducing intra-abdominal adiposity and reducing the inflammation associated with abdominal obesity. Insulin also exerts an anabolic effect of body fat distribution, favouring visceral adiposity in PCOS (Essah & Nestler, 2006).

The mechanism by which visceral adipose tissue contributes to insulin resistance is probably through increased release of free fatty acids by visceral fat due to suppression of lipolysis of subcutaneous tissue, which drains to the liver via the portal vein and obstructs insulin signaling, causing insulin resistance and hyperinsulinemia (Essah & Nestler, 2006). Weight loss in overweight or obese patients would have the additional benefit of reducing intra-abdominal adiposity and of correcting the pathologically altered adipokine secretion associated with abdominal obesity. In addition to this, insulin exerts an anabolic effect on body fat distribution, and is very likely to play a role in the development of visceral obesity in PCOS (Essah & Nestler, 2006).

Abdominal fat in PCOS can be measured by the waist-hip-ratio (WHR). For this measurement, the waistline circumference (WC) is simply divided by the hip circumference. This is, however, a crude measurement of visceral fat. Where more advanced imaging techniques were used, non-obese women with PCOS showed a higher percentage of total body fat in their upper body, and no difference in lower body fat compared with the controls (Sikaris, 2004). Even with modest weight loss (5% to 10% of original body weight), the reduction in visceral fat mass can be significant, which can lead to an improvement in metabolic parameters. Waist circumference (WC), *per se*, is a more accurate way of assessing reduction in visceral fat, as WHR and BMI have been shown to have poor correlation to visceral fat rating (Essah & Nestler, 2006; Norman et al., 2002).

Penaforte et al. (2011) used bio-electrical impedance (BI) to measure the weight, fat mass, and subcutaneous arm fat, together with trunk, neck and hip circumferences. Computed tomography (CT) was used to assess total abdominal fat, visceral fat and trunk fat (subcutaneous fat in the trunk + visceral fat). The study showed a good correlation between measured trunk circumference and assessment of trunk fat by CT. The researchers concluded that manually-measured trunk circumference holds close association with metabolic variables in PCOS and is a valuable tool for the assessment of body fat distribution in obese women with PCOS (Penaforte et al., 2011).

The existence of oxidative stress in PCOS is characterized by increased production of free radicals followed by decreased blood-antioxidant levels and has been demonstrated even in young, non-obese women with PCOS. The presence of oxidative stress exacerbates all the hormone imbalances in PCOS, and influences the ovarian theca cells, resulting in anovulation and CVD risk (Macut et al., 2017).

Factors such as reduced postprandial thermogenesis (the amount of energy expended after a meal had been eaten) might play a substantial role, as shown by Robinson et al. (1992). When compared to weight-matched controls, overweight PCOS women showed a reduction of 42kJ in postprandial thermogenesis. The researchers concluded that, if this reduction of energy expenditure should continue in the long term, a weight gain of 1.9 kg per year could be the result. These and other researchers did not find any difference in resting energy expenditure (REE) between weight-matched PCOS and non-PCOS women (Penaforte et al., 2009).

2.7. ABDOMINAL FAT-CELL DYSFUNCTION AND PCOS

Recently, the effects of improved lifestyle on female reproduction has been receiving attention. Focus has also been placed on the effects of BMI, nutritional intake and foods, physical activity and psychological stress on female reproduction. A central factor in the pathogenesis of PCOS might be dysfunctional fat cells, which contribute to insulin resistance and its consequences (Silvestris et al., 2018). Just like the HPO-axis, there seems to be a complex interaction between the pituitary gland, the pancreas, and the ovary, that results in an altered hormonal secretion pattern. When compared with BMI-matched controls, women with PCOS have a higher amount of visceral fat with a larger fat cell volume, and lower serum-adiponectin values (Arora, 2017).

In recent years, the physiology of infertility has been researched with regards to the dysfunction of adipose tissue, and the effects of the family of adipose-specific adipokines, secreted by adipose cells. These adipokines include leptin, adiponecin, resistin, visfatin and omentin, and as already mentioned, non-adipose specific cytokines such as tumour necrosis factor alpha (TNF-α) and interleukin-6 (IL-6). In PCOS, a severe dysfunction of adipose tissue has been noted, specifically the over-production of TNF-α, and the reduction of less inflammatory or "beneficial adipokines" such as adiponectin (Silvestris et al., 2018). An in-depth discussion of all the adipokines falls beyond the scope of this book, but leptin and adiponectin are briefly discussed hereafter.

2.7.1. Leptin

The first discovered adipokine to realize the endocrine function of adipose tissue, was leptin. Leptin is secreted in tandem with adipose mass, and is found in abundance in subjects with excessive abdominal fat. The actual function of leptin is to suppress food intake and enhance energy expenditure via direct effects on hypothalamic neurons. Leptin is thus considered an anorexigenic or anti-obesity hormone, and its levels increase after food intake, and decrease with fasting (Silvestris et al., 2018). The leptin receptor (LEPR) becomes down-regulated in the brain of obese women with very high circulating levels of leptin, also known as leptin resistance. Lower rates of pregnancy through IVF have been reported in females with higher leptin/BMI ratios.

In obese women with normal menstrual cycles, LH pulsality was significantly lower, thereby suggesting a hypothalamic defect. The higher levels of leptin found in obese women also compare with high levels of leptin found in the follicular fluid. This detrimental effect of increased leptin in obesity on the physiology of the oocyte, could lead to downstream effects, such as poor endometrial receptivity and embryo implantation (Silvestris et al., 2018).

2.7.2. Adiponectin

Adiponectin, a hormone secreted by fat cells, seems to exert a protective effect against insulin resistance, diabetes and cardiovascular disease, and seems to inhibit androgen production by the theca cells of the ovarian follicle. Reduced adiponectin directly influences the ovarian tissue and androgen production by the theca cells in females with PCOS. This is another example of a direct link between obesity and increased androgen production in women with PCOS, over and above the effect of IR (Arora, 2017). In this way, lower levels of circulating adiponectin found in PCOS women could play a distinct role in the pathogenesis of IR in women with PCOS (Macut et al., 2017).

Adiponectin ameliorates LH and GnRH, showing that it possibly plays a role in modulating the HPO-axis. Adiponectin levels decrease with obesity and increase with weight loss, and the main attributes of adiponectin are its ability to increase insulin sensitivity, and decrease triglyceride accumulation. Compared with fertile women, reduced adiponectin levels have been observed in women with recurrent implantation failure, in comparison with fertile women. This suggests the importance of adiponectin signaling in endometrial receptivity and its possible contribution to implantation failures and pregnancy loss in obese women with or without PCOS (Silvestris et al., 2018).

2.8. NUTRITION-RELATED FACTORS RELEVANT TO OVARIAN DYSFUNCTION

2.8.1. Nutrient Excess

The human body has an extraordinary capacity to maintain stable blood sugar levels and avoid swings in blood sugar. This capacity includes the hormones that are directly or indirectly generated by the dietary intake, sensing dietary nutrients, and relaying neural signals to the hypothalamus to orchestrate incoming fuel either for energy usage, or long-term storage. The central hormone involved in this communication is insulin. Inflammation disturbs this communication system, leading to metabolic defects such as obesity, diabetes, metabolic syndrome and PCOS. While insulin is the primary regulator of carbohydrate, fat, and protein metabolism, and indicates the metabolic availability of the different fuels to the brain, is it kept within a therapeutic concentration, critical for survival (Sears & Perry, 2015).

Our modern concern is not access to adequate nutrients as in the case of our ancestors, but rather one of excess nutrient intake. In this regard, insulin plays a central role in body defences against potential damage, by using adipose tissue, liver, and skeletal muscle as biological buffers against excessive nutrient intake.

All nutrients naturally have an inflammatory effect, since their conversion into energy or other biological materials generate responses that activate inflammation. This necessarily means that the intake of excess nutrients sets the scene for the generation of excess inflammation, whereby the ability of insulin to regulate metabolism, becomes compromised (Sears & Perry, 2015).

2.8.1.1. Adipose Tissue

The definition of obesity is an excess of body fat. Obesity is different from insulin resistance, in that it is not necessarily an adverse condition, provided that the fat is safely stored in healthy fat cells, which respond to the actions of insulin. As earlier described (Section 2.2), IR is a condition where cells no longer show appropriate response to insulin (Sears & Perry, 2015).

Insulin resistance appears to start in the hypothalamus. The arcuate nucleus in the hypothalamus acts to match satiety signals with adiposity, and blood-hormonal signals with hunger and food intake. Excessive nutritional intake (and especially saturated fat) causes inflammation of the hypothalamus, and deregulation of hunger and satiety signals. Especially the signaling of the satiety-inducing hormone leptin (see Section 2.12.3) is blunted through resistance, and as a result satiety is decreased and hunger increases. As hunger increases, excess dietary intake ensues (Sear & Perry).

The fat cells are the only cells in the body that are designed to safely store large amounts of fat as triglyceride, in which fatty acids are bound to a glycerol backbone. There are no adverse effects to the person carrying excess fat, as long as the fat cells are healthy and sensitive towards insulin, and these "metabolically-healthy obese" individuals make up roughly one third of the obese population. However, fat cells do not have an unlimited capacity to expand, and the over-expansion of the fat cells results in hypoxia (decreased oxygen supply), release of highly inflammatory factors inside the fat cell, and cell death. In turn, this creates insulin resistance within the fat cell and an influx of neutrophils and macrophages to clear the cellular debris. In the light of these events, insulin is no longer able to prevent fat release, and higher levels of free fatty acids (FFA), which result from dismantled triglycerides, leave the fat cell to enter the circulation, where they are taken up by the liver and skeletal muscles, which are unable to safely store large amounts of fat. The production of fat-binding proteins increases, to bind the newly-released FFA and take them into fat cells for storage. The increased flux of FFA in and out of the fat tissue creates a vicious cycle in which insulin resistance creates greater hunger, via malfunction in the hypothalamus (Sears & Perry, 2015).

Fatty tissue is rich in stem cells, and theoretically, should be able to produce new, healthy fat cells within the adipose tissue, but inflammatory factors (such as TNF-α) inhibit this. The inability to form new fat cells and the continuous expansion of existing fats cells, accelerate fat cell death and adipose tissue inflammation. Once the fat cells become unable to deal with the increasing fatty acid flow, the excess begins to accumulate in other organs, such as the liver and skeletal muscle, the cells of which are unable to store large amounts of fat safely. Thus, begins the process of lipotoxicity, which accelerates the consequences of insulin resistance (Sears & Perry, 2015). Lipotoxicity has been cited for its oocyte damage, as well as production of weak embryos, and implantation difficulty in overweight females (Silvestris, 2018).

2.8.1.2. Reproduction

The increased flux of FFA also causes damage to non-adipose cells, by increasing the free radicals in the body, inducing stress and death of multiple cell types, including oocytes. The inflammation caused by FFA can be substantiated by circulating levels of CRP and triglycerides. The link between obesity and miscarriage has also been studied repeatedly, where the risk of miscarriage in obese women has been found as high as 40%, as opposed to 15% in females of normal weight. Overweight and obese women also have poorer outcomes after fertility treatment, compared to normal-weight women. Overweight and obese women show a poor response to ovulation induction, require higher doses of gonadotropins, and need longer treatment duration for follicle development and ovulation. The oocyte yield is lower, and the rate of cycle cancellation is higher in obese women. Their assisted reproduction technology procedures yield fewer follicles, with a poor follicular harvest (Silvestris et al., 2018).

Obesity is pathogenically associated with inflammation, and all mechanisms which are necessary for normal oocyte development, are deregulated. Since the major mechanisms that regulate the normal activities of the female reproductive system are deranged in the face of adipose excess, obesity is now recognized as a direct opposition to female fertility, through the HPO-axis (Silvestris et al., 2018).

2.8.1.3. Liver

Unlike adipose tissue, the liver cannot safely store excessive fat. The build-up of fatty deposits in the liver is one of the first adverse metabolic consequences of insulin resistance, and is referred to as non-alcoholic fatty liver disease (NAFLD) (Sears & Perry, 2015).

2.8.1.4. Pancreas

The β-cells of the pancreas sense glucose levels in the blood via glucokinase, and secrete insulin in response. The pancreatic β-cells are not normally prone to insulin resistance, but highly prone to toxicity from inflammatory agents, such as the metabolites of arachidonic acid (AA), the inflammatory end-product of omega-6 fats. With damage to the β-cells the pancreas is no longer able to maintain adequate levels of insulin secretion to clear blood glucose levels to normal, and the development of T2DM becomes rapid (Sears & Perry, 2015).

2.8.2. Nutrition-Induced Inflammation

As already mentioned (Section 1.6), PCOS is characterized not only by ovarian dysfunction, but hyperandrogenism and polycystic morphology of the ovaries. Of the four phenotypes generated by the Rotterdam criteria, three have hyperandrogenism as a feature, especially "classic" PCOS. This is of key importance as hyperandrogenism is strongly implicated in the aetiology of PCOS and connected with the metabolic derangements that underlie the pathology. The pro-inflammatory character of PCOS is well established, and recent evidence points towards nutrient-induced oxidative stress and inflammation as a cause of the metabolic and ovarian dysfunctions. Furthermore, overwhelming evidence shows that in PCOS, hyperandrogenism is linked to inflammation, and this has prompted further research in the field. Data is emerging that nutrient-induced inflammation might directly be responsible for the excess production of androgens by the ovaries (González, 2015).

With the finding of high levels of TNF-α in both overweight and normal-weight PCOS women, the notion that PCOS is a pro-inflammatory state was confirmed. Several pro-inflammatory markers have been associated with PCOS, including TNF-α, IL-6, and CRP.

C-reactive protein (CRP) has been shown to be the most reliable marker of inflammation in PCOS. Normal-weight PCOS women demonstrate elevated CRP levels, but lower than that of non-PCOS overweight women, suggesting that CRP levels due to PCOS is obscured in the presence of obesity, but still high enough in PCOS women of normal weight to pose a substantial cardiovascular risk. The enlarged adipose tissue compartment of the obese woman creates a pro-inflammatory environment which, added to PCOS, increases the severity of the metabolic abnormalities of PCOS *per se* (González, 2015).

In PCOS women, the insulin receptor has no genetic or functional abnormalities, and as in the case of obesity, the cause of insulin resistance in PCOS is found to be a post-receptor defect in insulin signaling. Evidence also points to the probability that the inflammatory capabilities of TNF-α is what mediates insulin resistance in PCOS women (González, 2015).

In the 1980s, the dogma was born that the compensatory hyperinsulinemia of insulin resistance promotes hyperandrogenism in PCOS. These studies were done almost exclusively on obese PCOS women, and hyperandrogenism could only be elicited with supra-physiological insulin infusions. Insulin infused in physiological doses, to the contrary, has no effect on androgen levels in PCOS, so the dogma also does not explain the cause of hyperandrogenism in the 30% of females with PCOS without insulin resistance or those of normal weight. This raises the possibility that inflammation may directly induce hyperandrogenism in PCOS (González, 2015).

Data showing the inflammatory capabilities of glucose and saturated fat, have provided further insight into the cause of IR and atherogenesis in PCOS. Glucose and saturated fat in PCOS, stimulate an inflammatory response, which is manifested by increased free radicals and oxidative stress, and the activation of the *cardinal signal of inflammation*, nuclear factor kappa-B (NF-kB), all of which happens independent of obesity. Nutrient-induced inflammation thus leads to pro-inflammatory signaling, known to cause IR and atherogenesis in PCOS (González, 2015).

It has already been mentioned that women with PCOS have a five-fold to ten-fold higher risk of developing T2DM, compared with non-PCOS women of similar weight and age (Essah & Nestler, 2006). The progressive deterioration of pancreatic β-cell function eventually leads to a rise in circulating glucose, and in susceptible individuals culminates in β-cell failure and T2DM. Oxidative stress and inflammation from hyperglycemia further exacerbate the degeneration of β-cells.

A link has been established between β-cell dysfunction and inflammation in PCOS. Upon initial glucose ingestion, there is a readily available pool of insulin in the β-cell (first phase), which is followed by synthesis of new insulin to manage glucose fluctuations after the meal (second phase). Women with PCOS of normal weight have mild disturbance of the first phase β-cell function, where obese women with PCOS exhibit disturbances in both first and second phase β-cell function. First phase β-cell dysfunction generates free radicals and oxidative stress, as well as release of TNF-α secretion, where first and second phase β-cell dysfunction further causes NF-kB activation and elevated circulating CRP levels. From these findings, it becomes clear that in PCOS, nutrient-induced oxidative stress and inflammation play a direct role in the deterioration of β-cell function prior to development of overt hyperglycemia, which is worsened by concomitant obesity (González, 2015).

To summarize, although hyperandrogenism precedes the pro-inflammatory state of PCOS, it is not the major contributor. Recent data points to inflammation as the direct stimulator of excess ovarian androgen production. The inflammation caused by excess glucose and saturated fat is capable of the metabolic derangements and ovarian dysfunction in PCOS women, and is exacerbated by the added inflammation by the presence of obesity (González, 2015).

2.8.3. Advanced Glycation End-Products (AGEs)

The end-products of a chemical procedure which involves the non-enzymatical reaction between carbohydrates (sugars), fats and proteins, also known as the Maillard reaction, are termed 'advanced glycation end-products' (AGEs) and known as glycotoxins (Garg & Merhi, 2016; Uribarri et al., 2015).

In the early stage of this process, the glycosylated products are reversible, also known as Schiff-base and Amadori products. The Amadori products undergo dehydration and re-arrangements, leading to the late-stage Maillard reaction, which is irreversible. The significance of AGEs formed in this way, with regards to mediating diabetic complications and aging, was only recognized in the 1980s. The reversible Schiff-base products are formed through glycation (as opposed to enzymatically glycosylated proteins), and in the end stage, the complex pigments and cross links formed during the Maillard reaction, form glycated proteins, are known as AGEs (see Figure 7) (Merhi, 2014).

AGEs can also be generated by several other reactions, including the oxidation of sugars, fats, and amino acids, to create reactive compounds that bind to proteins (Uribarri et al., 2015). A classic example of the Maillard reaction in the culinary world is the formation of browned caramel from sweetened condensed milk, after application of moist heat for a long time. The Maillard reaction is also used to brown food such as frying, broiling, or applying direct heat to create browning and enhanced taste, such as the toasting of bread and deep-frying of foods in which starch and sugar are combined, for example donuts and other bakery products.

AGEs might well contribute to the aetiology and pathogenesis of PCOS, since they are one of the emerging pro-inflammatory molecules that have been found to be elevated in PCOS. There might also be a relationship between elevated AGE levels and ovarian reserve in females of reproductive age (Merhi, 2015; Pertynska-Marczewska et al., 2015).

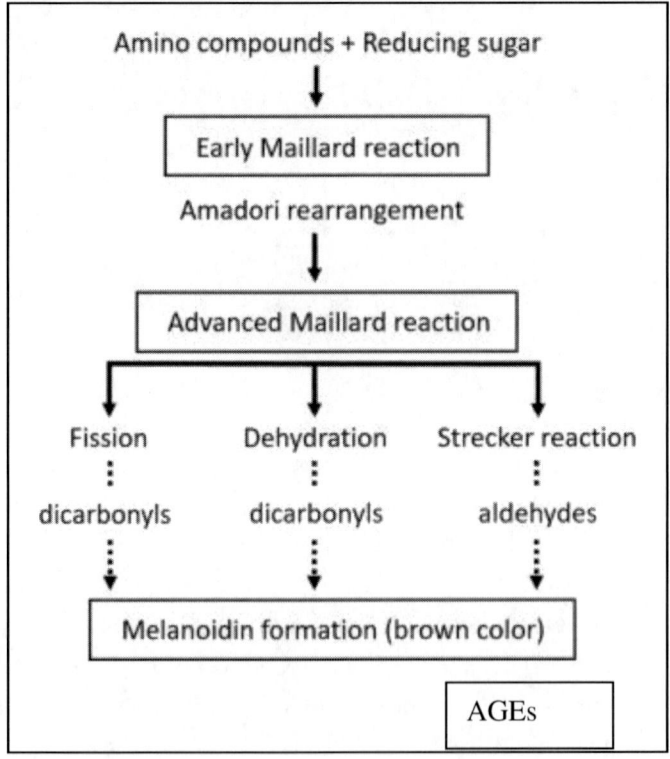

Source: Arihara, Zhou & Ohata, 2017.

Figure 7. The steps in the Maillard reaction.

In October 2014, researchers met in Mexico to discuss the potential role of dietary AGEs, since awareness had increased about the substantial contribution by these substances to increase oxidative stress and inflammation, playing a major role in causing chronic disease. The full report of this meeting falls outside of the scope of this book, but sufficient understanding of the biochemical action of AGEs is necessary to value the extent of their detriment and cellular damage as well as the dietary recommendations to reduce AGE consumption.

AGEs are produced slowly in the human body, being accelerated by oxidative stress, insulin resistance, hyperglycemia, aging and several other factors. Elevated levels of AGEs which accumulate in time are associated with T2DM, MS and related conditions, and aging, including accelerated ovarian aging. Elevated levels of AGEs are even considered an aetiological factor in PCOS (Merhi, 2014).

The cell receptor for AGEs is referred to as RAGE, situated on the extracellular matrix. AGEs may also exert their action independent of RAGE, through cross-linking with other cell receptors. When AGEs link with RAGE (AGE-RAGE), the interaction leads to activation of NF-kB, and development of a pro-inflammatory state, cellular toxicity and damage, and apoptosis (cell death).

RAGE is found in abundance in many organs, such as the heart, lungs, skeletal muscle and blood vessels, but also on the ovaries (Merhi, 2014). Free radicals and oxidative stress caused by RAGE activation, leads to a positive feedback loop, whereby RAGE expression is up-regulated, leading to exacerbation of inflammatory processes. RAGE expression has recently been linked to the development of PCOS, as one of the inflammatory processes (Merhi, 2014; Pertynska-Marczewska et al., 2015). Women with PCOS have elevated levels of AGEs, and also show increased expression of RAGE in the ovarian tissue.

There is another receptor for AGEs, which does not have a trans-membrane basis, and is found in circulating blood. These receptors are known as soluble RAGE (sRAGE). These AGE receptors are regarded as "good" receptors, as they are able to bind AGEs in circulation and act as a decoy, preventing AGEs from binding to RAGE. Soluble RAGE is often regarded as an anti-inflammatory receptor (Merhi, 2014; Pertynska-Marczewska et al., 2015).

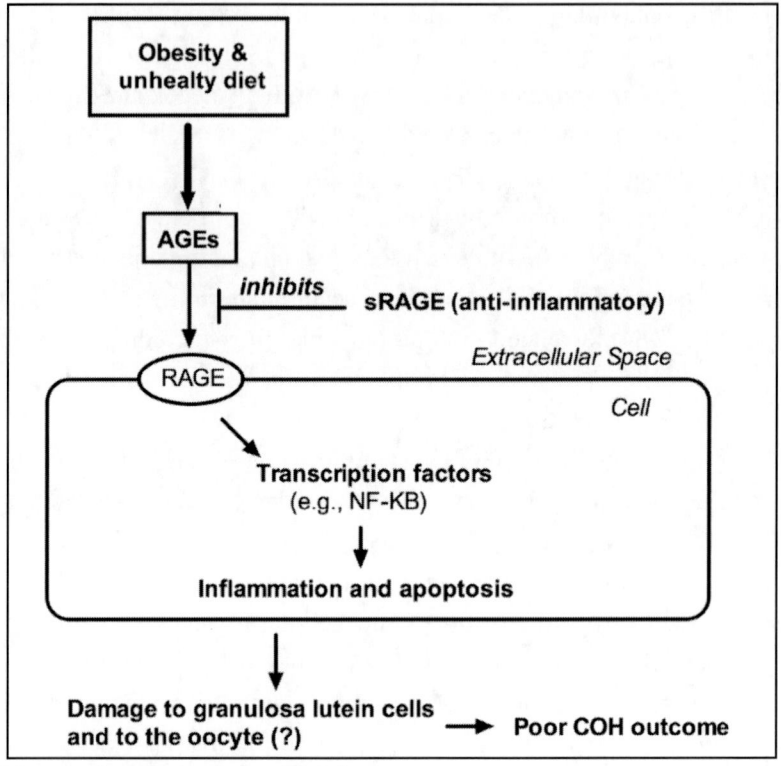

* COH: controlled ovarian hyperstimulation.
Source: Adapted from Zhang & Merhi, 2016.

Figure 8. The AGE-RAGE interaction.

Serum levels of AGEs have been found to correlate with the hormonal abnormalities such as those seen in PCOS, and a distinct correlation between levels of AGEs and testosterone has been shown. It is also known that changes in dietary AGEs are related to changes in insulin sensitivity, oxidative stress and other hormones in women with PCOS, so that these variables may be significantly improved by reducing the number of dietary AGEs. The improvement on insulin sensitivity seen in a study on women with PCOS eating a low-AGE diet, over those on a high-AGE diet was significant. Consequently, the researchers strongly suggested that dietary habits play a large role in the pathology of PCOS. The improved effects on a low-AGEs diet were seen independent of changes in BMI (Pertynska-Marczewska et al., 2015).

The levels of AGEs in the body are influenced both by endogenous and exogenous factors. AGEs can be endogenously formed as a consequence of high dietary sugar intake (an example of such is glycosylated haemoglobin A1C (HbA1C), a marker of diabetic glycemic control over a period of three months), while exogenous AGEs are ingested by high temperature processed foods, inhalation of tobacco smoking or use of tobacco products, and trace metals. Two large databases are available for use to estimate dietary intake of AGEs and to change dietary habit and make better choices to reduce the intake of AGEs. Knowledge about different culinary techniques that reduce the amount of AGEs in the end product, without changing the type and quality of the foods consumed, may be of valuable help (Ubarri et al., 2015).

Table 2 gives a short summary of food containing high and low AGEs. Methods such as steaming and stewing of meat, where use is made of moist heat, will generate much less AGEs than the other methods already mentioned, such as frying, grilling, broiling or searing. Lowering the pH of food (e.g. by marinating) may contribute to reducing the AGEs content of foods (Uribarri et al., 2015).

Table 2. Examples of foods containing high and low AGEs

High AGEs		Low AGEs	
Food item	AGEs	Food item	AGEs
Beef, fried	9 522	Beef, stewed	2 443
Chicken, roasted	5 975	Chicken, broiled	2 232
Beef frankfurter, broiled	10 143	Beef frankfurter, boiled	6 736
Lamb, broiled	2 188	Lamb, boiled	1 096
Salmon, broiled	3 012	Salmon, poached	2 063
Potato, French fried	694	Potato, boiled	17

Note: AGE content of foods expressed in arbitrary AGE kilounits per 90g serving for meats, and 100g serving for potatoes.
Source: Uribarri et al., 2010.

The elevated AGEs correspond to enhanced expression of RAGE in ovarian tissue, and also increased ovarian weight, fasting glucose, insulin and testosterone levels in animal studies. Human studies on diabetics showed a significant reduction of circulating AGEs with dietary restriction, and showed improved insulin sensitivity and stabilized progression of atherosclerosis (Mehri, 2015). Should the exact mechanism by which AGEs induce hyperandrogenism in PCOS be established, the targeted therapy will greatly enhance the reproductive outcome in this population (Garg & Merhi, 2016).

Research has clearly shown that infertility and anovulation are associated with obesity, and studies have suggested that oocyte quantity and quality is an important factor in obese women seeking conception through assisted reproductive technology (ART). Because obese women have elevated levels of AGEs, oocyte competency might be negatively affected during controlled ovarian hyperstimulation (COH) for procedures of ART. Literature from ART studies as cited by Garg & Merhi (2016) have shown that higher levels of AGEs in the serum and follicular fluid negatively correlated with follicular growth and oocyte fertilization, indicating reduced fertility. Another study showed the presence of AGE-modified proteins on the surface of freshly-harvested human granulosa cells from women who underwent COH. This implies that AGEs may be involved in the decline of ovarian function, and that women with higher levels of AGEs, such as obese women, might have a poorer response to COH (Zhang & Merhi, 2016).

The modern diet is a strong contributor to the circulating levels of AGEs in the human body, and has a significant impact on health and disease. A review by Aragno and Mastrocola (2017) highlighted the finding that fructose is more active than glucose in generating glycation precursors, possibly contributing to AGE formation, especially in the light of the modern higher fructose intake, as compared with decades ago. Sustained exposure to exogenous AGEs, which are highly pro-oxidant, gradually erodes natural defences. This in turn creates abnormally-high levels of free radicals and inflammation, which place a high burden on the immune system and precedes diseases, amongst others, diabetes and CVD, but also premature ageing and depletion of ovarian reserves.

A very simple intervention is accessible in the form of an AGEs-controlled diet, which has been shown to be feasible and safe. In 2010, Uribarri and colleagues published an extended list of foods with their AGEs content, which serves as a practical guide to decrease the AGEs content of the daily dietary intake. However, much more research in the field of AGEs in health and disease is necessary to answer many yet unresolved issues and questions (Ubarri et al., 2015).

Interestingly, a recent article in the Indian Journal of Endocrinology and Metabolism (Tanguturi & Nagarakanti, 2018) described how the AGEs-induced oxidative stress in PCOS subjects, exposed them to increased risk of periodontal disease, causing oxidative stress in the gingival with accelerated tissue damage. In the presence of gingival inflammation, the hormonal changes in PCOS might affect the salivary defences to bacteria, since the accumulation of progesterone and estrogen in periodontal tissues are capable of providing a favourable growth environment for bacteria (Tanguturi & Nagarakanti, 2018).

2.8.4. Trans Fats

Very little research had been done on the effect of different fats on female reproduction, until 2007. Chavarro et al. (2007b) conducted a trial lasting 8 years, including 18 500 subjects, and examined the association between the intakes of different types of fat and ovulatory infertility. The results revealed that intakes of cholesterol, saturated fat, mono-unsaturated fat, and total poly-unsaturated fats (Ω-3 plus Ω-6 fats) were unrelated to ovulatory infertility, but that there was a significant positive link between trans-fat consumption and infertility-risk.

Daily energy intake above two percent (2%) of the total, in the form of trans fat, was associated with a 73% greater risk of ovulatory infertility. Age, smoking, parity, use of oral contraceptives in the past, BMI, length of menstrual cycle and presence of androgen excess did not make any difference to the results. Intake of trans-fatty acids is also associated with increased concentrations of inflammatory markers, and with greater insulin resistance and risk for type-2 diabetes mellitus which adversely affect ovulatory function.

High intake of trans-fatty acids was also found to indicate less health consciousness, which is of concern in couples who are seeking fertility. Women planning to become pregnant should receive advice regarding their fat intake to improve their overall risk for CVD and diabetes, although responding well to such advice could improve their fertility as well (Chavarro et al., 2008).

Although most fats originate from either plants or animals, trans fats are industrial fats, and by-products of a chemical reaction known as hydrogenation. Hydrogen gas is bubbled through the liquid oil under high pressure, together with a catalyst, to form a solid fat out of a fluid oil, in order to make it semi-solid, and extend its lifespan and reduce its degeneration or oxidation during repeated heat-application. This process is known as partial hydrogenation. Should the hydrogenation process be applied in full, the resultant fat would be completely saturated, hard and unspreadable, which is one of the characteristics that make margarine (partially hydrogenated vegetable oil) attractive – it can be taken from the refrigerator and spread easily even if cold.

Peroxisome proliferator-activated receptors (PPARs) are transcription factors of nuclear hormone receptors, a superfamily comprising of the following three subtypes: PPAR-α, PPAR-γ, and PPAR-β/δ. Activation of PPAR-α reduces triglyceride level and is involved in energy homeostasis. Activation of PPAR-γ causes insulin sensitivity and regulates glucose metabolism, whereas activation of PPAR-β/δ enhances fat metabolism. The PPAR family of nuclear receptors plays a major regulatory role in energy regulation and metabolic function. PPAR antagonists play a large role in causing dyslipidemia, diabetes, fat cell dysfunction, inflammation, infertility or dysfunctional reproduction, and obesity (Tyagi et al., 2011).

The activation of PPAR-γ is a beneficial process to human health, and trans fats do the opposite – they suppress PPAR-γ. In 2008, it was estimated that the amount of trans fat in the average American diet was 6g per day, which reduces the beneficial effect of activated PPAR-γ by 50%. This also means that IR increases, with resultant reduction in fertility. Concomitantly, trans fats elevate inflammation throughout the body, interfering with ovulation, conception, and early embryonic development (Chavarro et al., 2008). Furthermore, as PPAR-γ plays an essential role in placental maturation, function, and hormone production, trans fats might promote the risk of pregnancy loss through suppression of PPAR-γ.

Morrison, Glueck and Wang (2008) researched the association between dietary intake of trans fat and fetal loss, and found a significant, curvi-linear, independent relationship between caloric intake from trans fats, and fetal loss. The overall risk of fetal loss increased as the percentage of caloric intake from trans fats increased, with a sharp increase in fetal loss when the intake of trans fats superceded 4.7% of caloric intake (Morrison et al., 2008).

The National Academy of Sciences (NAS) advises the governments of the United States of America (USA) and Canada on nutritional science, for use in public policy and product labeling programs. Their 2002 *Dietary Reference Intakes for Energy, Carbohydrate, Fiber, Fat, Fatty Acids, Cholesterol, Protein, and Amino Acids* presented their findings, suggestions, and recommendations regarding consumption of trans fat (Trumbo et al., 2002). They based their recommendations on two key facts: Firstly, "trans fatty acids are not essential and provide no known benefit to human health", whether of plant or animal origin. Secondly, while both saturated and trans fats have been shown to raise levels of LDL, trans fats also reduce levels of HDL, thus, increasing the risk of cardiovascular disease. The NAS indicated concern "that dietary trans fatty acids are more deleterious with respect to coronary artery disease than saturated fatty acids".

This was supported by a 2006 New England Journal of Medicine (NEJM) scientific review that stated: "...from a nutritional standpoint, the consumption of trans fatty acids results in considerable potential harm but no apparent benefit" (Mozaffarian et al., 2006).

In the light of these facts and concerns, the NAS concluded that there is no safe level of trans-fat consumption. Moreover, there is no adequate level, recommended daily amount or tolerable upper limit for trans fats. This is because any incremental increase in trans-fat intake likewise increases the risk of coronary artery disease and other diseases.

A very small amount of trans fats are present in the products of ruminant animals, but the US National Dairy Council has asserted that these trans fats present in animal products are of a different nature than those in partially-hydrogenated oils, and do not appear to exhibit the same negative effects. A recent scientific review agrees with the conclusion that: "the sum of the current evidence suggests that the Public health implications of consuming trans fats from ruminant products are relatively limited" (Mozaffarian et al., 2006). Like the NAS, the World Health Organization has attempted to balance public health goals with a practical level of trans-fat consumption, recommending in 2003 that trans fats be limited to less than one percent (1%) of overall energy intake (Field, 2006).

Trans fats have been found to be such a potent deterrent to fertility, that bans have been placed on trans fats in commercial products, by several countries and institutions. Until 2006, labels referred to trans fats as "partially-hydrogenated vegetable oils" or "vegetable shortening", which were terms only recognized by the informed consumer. In January 2006, legislation in the USA changed, requiring food labels to reveal the trans-fat content amongst the content of other fats, such as saturated and unsaturated fat (Chavarro et al., 2008).

Until the early 1900s, the only sources of trans fats were the bacteria in the stomachs of ruminants, such as cows, sheep, deer, buffalo, venison and dairy products, in very small amounts. Until then, they were also the only source of trans fat that humans could consume. Today, trans fats are widespread, and used especially for their properties of food and condiment preservation, as they have a long shelf life, and they can be heated over and over without turning rancid. Examples of such foods are margarines, vegetable shortening, packaged cookies and other baked goods, donuts, fast-food potato chips or French fries.

The type of trans fat that occurs naturally in the milk and body fat of ruminants at a level of two to five percent (2 to 5%) of total fat, are natural trans fats, which include conjugated linoleic acid (CLA). CLA has two double bonds, one in the *cis* configuration and one in *trans*, which makes it simultaneously a *cis*- and a *trans*-fatty acid, and cannot be viewed as solely a trans fat. Some evidence exists that CLA might have beneficial properties in several health issues, including heart disease, cancer, and obesity (Field, 2006).

2.8.5. Fructose: The Effect of Excessive Fructose Consumption on the Development of Insulin Resistance and Metabolic Syndrome

Insulin resistance has often been linked to the macronutrient content of the diet, and, in the past, diets high in saturated fats have been shown to induce weight gain, IR and hyperlipidemia in both animals and humans. Several recent reviews agree in their conclusion that, while there is strong evidence that diets high in fructose can produce obesity, IR/glucose intolerance and dyslipidemia in animals, direct experimental evidence that chronic consumption of fructose promotes the development of the MS in humans is equivocal (Basciano, Federico & Adeli, 2005, Elliott et al., 2002, Havel, 2005, Stanhope & Havel, 2008).

2.8.5.1. Differences in Metabolic Pathways of Glucose and Fructose

Key differences in the metabolic pathways that glucose and fructose follow are apparent (Figure 9). The ability of the liver to metabolise high doses of fructose is believed to be responsible for the disruption in energy stores and fuel metabolism that is observed in excessive fructose intake. Of key importance is the ability of fructose to bypass the main regulatory step in glycolysis, namely the conversion of glucose-6-phosphate to fructose 1.6-biphosphate, which is controlled by phosphofructokinase (PFK). Thus, while glucose metabolism is negatively regulated by PFK, fructose can continuously enter the glycolytic pathway, uncontrollably producing glucose, glycogen, lactate, and pyruvate, providing both the glycerol and acetyl portions of triglyceride molecules (Basciano et al., 2005; Lê & Tappy, 2006). The bypass can also result in increased glycogen deposition and in de novo lipogenesis (DNL) (Elliott et al., 2002, Vos et al., 2008, Lê & Tappy, 2006).

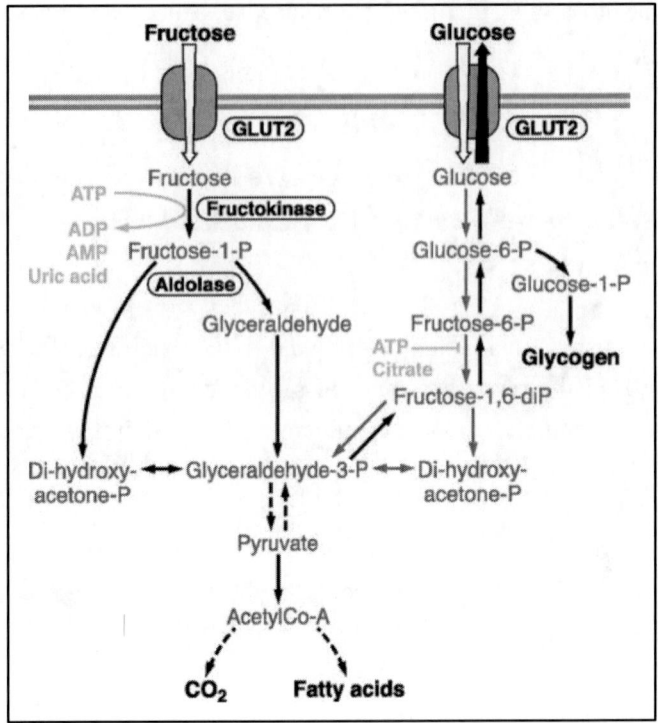

Source: Tappy & Lê, 2010.

Figure 9. Different hepatic pathways of fructose and glucose.

Other differences are present in the metabolism of fructose and glucose. The transport mechanism of glucose into cells is known as glucose transporter type-4 (GLUT-4), and is insulin-dependent in most tissues. Once insulin has activated the insulin receptor, the density of glucose transporters on the cell surface rapidly increases, and facilitates entry of glucose into the cell. Next, glucose is phosphorylated to glucose-6-phosphate by glucokinase, and the intracellular metabolism of glucose begins. Through modulation by phosphofructokinase, the conversion of glucose-6-phosphate to the glycerol backbone of triglycerides can be tightly controlled. As opposed to glucose, fructose is transported into hepatic cells via a non-insulin dependent mechanism, glucose transporter type-5 (GLUT-5). No GLUT-5 transporters are present in brain tissue and in the beta cells of the pancreas, indicating limited entry of fructose into the tissues concerned

(Bray, Nielsen & Popkin., 2004; Elliott et al., 2002; Havel, 2005). Previous studies have indicated that fructose, unlike glucose, at most has a weak ability to stimulate insulin from the beta cells of the pancreas (Stanhope & Havel, 2008). If fructose is given as part of a mixed meal, the rise in serum-glucose and insulin levels is smaller than, should an equal amount of glucose have been given (Bray et al., 2004).

The fructose-specific hexose transporter, GLUT-5, is primarily expressed in the jejunum on both the brush border and on the basolateral enterocyte membranes, as well as in the lower levels in the kidney, skeletal muscle and adipocytes. In the case of large fructose consumption, the capacity of GLUT-5 to absorb fructose is exceeded, and diarrhea can result. Intake of glucose together with fructose, as it should usually be consumed in beverages and with meals, seems to enhance fructose absorption. Some adaptation to high fructose intake takes place, as fructose absorption is increased during sustained high fructose intake (Havel, 2005).

2.8.5.2. Fructose Contents of Different Sources

Sucrose (table sugar) consists of 50% glucose and 50% fructose, with the latter not being an essential sugar for the human body. The percentage of fructose in high-fructose corn syrup (HFCS) used in sweetened beverages and sports drinks can be substantial, since HFCS contains between 42%, 55% and 90% fructose (HFCS-42, HFCS-55, and HFCS-90) (Basciano et al., 2005; Bray et al., 2004; Havel, 2005).

Although produced and widely used in many countries worldwide, the use of HFCS increased with 1000% in the United States between 1970 and 1990, with the country concerned being the largest user of HFCS worldwide (Basciano et al., 2005; Bray et al., 2004). Scant data exists on foods containing HFCS, other than in the USA. The starch in corn can be effectively converted to glucose and from there to various amounts of fructose, using a glucose isomerase. Corn-based syrups are inexpensive and have made it more profitable to replace sucrose and other simple sugars with HFCS, which now represents up to 40 to 43% of added caloric sweetener in the USA, being largely used in soft drinks and other sweetened beverages (Bray et al., 2004).

The sweetness of fructose is 1.73 times more than that of sucrose. If, for comparative purposes, the sweetness of sucrose is set at 100, the sweetness of glucose is 74. Replacing sucrose with HFCS in soft drinks impacts on the ratio of fructose to glucose, as HFCS-55 has a fructose to glucose ratio of 1.22, with 10% more fructose, by weight, than sucrose. Estimations are that 60% of the HFCS used in sweetened beverages comes from HFCS-55 and 40% from HFCS-42. In the combined use of sucrose, HFCS-55 and HFCS-42, the average fructose content of sweetened beverages can reasonably be approximated at 50% (Bray et al., 2004; Havel, 2005).

Crystalline fructose with a purity of 100% is also used to sweeten some foods and beverages, but scant data on the use of crystalline fructose is available (Havel, 2005). Together with the use of sucrose as added sweetener, it could be estimated that the total intake of added fructose, plus naturally-occurring fructose in fruit and fruit juices, is as much as 12% of total energy intake per day (Vos et al., 2008). This estimate includes consumption of not only sweetened beverages, fruit and fruit juices, but also sweets and desserts. Based on a daily energy intake of 2 000 calories per day, the fructose intake would be estimated as being at least 60g/day. Actual consumption of fructose is likely to be underestimated, due to selective underreporting of specific foods and drinks (Havel, 2005; Vos et al., 2008) with certain population groups in the USA likely consuming well over 100g fructose daily from added sweeteners (Havel, 2005).

Fruit juices differ widely in their content of fructose, with apple juice containing more than 60% of its caloric content in the form of fructose, and orange juice only 40 to 45%. Apple- and other juice-sweetened juices and beverages contain higher amounts of fructose as a percentage of the total caloric content than do soft drinks sweetened with HFCS-42 or HFCS-55. An increasing number of beverages and juice products are being sweetened with apple and white grape juice, resulting in a higher number of calories being provided by fructose (Bray et al., 2004; Havel, 2005).

Important note: Fruits, fruit juices and fructose-dominant foods cannot be judged by the GI value assigned to them, as fructose is not released as glucose into the bloodstream, and hence does not register with a GI value. The GI value of these products is mainly the result of the glucose content, and care should be taken to view such products as favourable or preferable because of their lower GI value. The same principle applies to "natural" sweeteners such as honey, maple syrup, and yakon syrup.

Investigators have linked the consumption of particularly apple juice, because of its popularity, to overweight and obesity in children aged 2 to 5 years. In 1999, a study showed that the incidence of overweight in children who consumed more than 360ml of any fruit juice per day was significantly higher than it was in those who consumed less. The researchers suggested that the increase in body weight seemed to be related to apple juice only, which has a high content of fructose. Other consecutive studies refuted the findings, although a recent prospective cohort of Mediterranean adults showed a weak, but significant, association between weight gain and sweetened fruit juice consumption. Since fruit juice remains an important source of nutrition of vitamins and minerals for children, further research of the association between fruit juice consumption and weight gain is warranted (Malik, Schulze & Hu, 2006).

Table 3. Carbohydrate composition (%) of commercial sweeteners

Sugar	Fructose	Glucose	Other saccharides
HFCS-42	42	53	5
HFCS-55	55	45	0
HFCS-90	90	10	0
Sucrose	50	50	0
Honey	49	43	8
Apple juice	59	31	10
Orange juice	51	49	0

Source: Moeller et al, 2009.

2.8.6. Fructose: A Highly-Lipogenic Nutrient

When small amounts of glucose are infused into the portal vein, hepatic uptake of glucose improves, probably due to the stimulation of glucokinase. Glycogen synthesis is also stimulated by increased carbon flux, by means of glycogen synthase, and, apart from stimulating glycogen synthesis, the above also restores the ability of hyperglycaemia to regulate the production of glucose in the liver. Hence, small amounts of fructose seem to act in a catalytic way to improve hepatic glucose uptake and storage as glycogen, mainly because of the stimulation of hepatic glucokinase (Havel, 2005). The fact was verified in an oral glucose tolerance test (OGTT) in which 10% of the glucose (75g) was added as fructose (7.5g). The outcome showed favourable results in adults with type-2 diabetes mellitus, suggesting that limited amounts of fructose would be useful in improving glycemic control in type-2 diabetes mellitus (Elliott et al., 2002; Havel, 2005).

The liver is capable of metabolising fructose. For millennia, the human body has been given fructose to the amount of 16g to 20g per day from fresh fruit (Basciano et al., 2005). From Table 4, it should be clear that, apart from dried fruit such as figs, any three fresh fruits can be eaten on a daily basis, without exceeding the above-cited amount of 16g to 20g. Westernisation of diets has resulted in significant increases in added fructose, leading to typical daily consumptions of 85g to 100g per day (Basciano et al., 2005; Elliott et al., 2002).

In the study by Vos et al. (2008), determining the fructose intake amongst US children, adolescents and adults, the highest intake (72.8g/day) was found to take place amongst adolescents who were 12 to 18 years of age. The exposure of the liver to such large quantities of fructose leads to the stimulation of lipogenesis and to rapid triglyceride accumulation, which, in turn, contributes to reduced insulin sensitivity and to hepatic insulin resistance/glucose intolerance (Basciano et al., 2005).

In an interim report on an ongoing investigation that compared fructose and glucose intake of 25% of total energy through beverages, Stanhope and Havel (2008) found that, in particular, the high-fructose group showed development of three of the pathological characteristics of MS: dyslipidaemia; insulin resistance; and increased visceral adipose tissue. The researchers further reported that, in older adults, as well as in shorter-term studies in younger adults, hypertriglyceridemia seems to be the earliest metabolic perturbation following high-fructose consumption. Current literature provides considerable evidence in support of the ability of high-fructose diets to up-regulate the lipogenesis pathway, which, in turn, leads to increased triglyceride production (Basciano et al., 2005; Stanhope & Havel, 2008).

Table 4. Sugar content of selected common fruit and vegetables (g/100g)

Food item	Total carbohydrate	Free fructose	Free glucose	Sucrose	Fructose/ glucose ratio
Fruits					
Apple	13.8	5.9	2.4	2.1	2.0
Apricot	11.1	0.9	2.4	5.9	0.7
Banana	22.8	4.9	5.0	2.4	1.0
Fig, dried	63.9	22.9	24.8	0.07	0.93
Grapes	18.1	8.1	7.2	0.2	1.1
Peach	9.5	1.5	2.0	4.8	0.9
Pear	15.5	6.2	2.8	0.8	2.1
Pineapple	13.1	2.1	1.7	6.0	1.1
Plum	11.4	3.1	5.1	1.6	0.66
Vegetables					
Beet, red	9.6	0.1	0.1	6.5	1.0
Carrot	9.6	0.6	0.6	3.6	1.0
Corn, sweet	19.0	1.9	3.4	0.9	0.61
Red pepper, sweet	6.0	2.3	1.9	0.0	1.2
Onion, sweet	7.6	2.0	2.3	0.7	0.9
Sugar beet		0.5	1.0	16 – 17	1.0
Sugar cane		1.0	1.0	11 – 16	1.0
Sweet potato	20.1	0.7	1.0	2.5	0.9

Source: Park & Yetley, 1973.

The most likely cause of postprandial hypertriglyceridemia is increased hepatic DNL, which stimulates very-low-density lipoprotein (VLDL) production and exit from the liver. Hepatic lipogenesis is promoted by high-fructose consumption in three ways:

- Fructose is mainly metabolised in the liver.

- Fructose enters into the glycolysis pathway via fructose-1-phosphate and hence bypasses the main rate-controlling step of glycolysis catalysed by phosphofructokinase, providing unregulated amounts of acetyl coenzyme A (acetyl-CoA) and glycerol-3-phosphate, which are both lipogenic substrates (Basciano et al., 2005; Elliott et al., 2002; Stanhope & Havel, 2008).
- Fructose is able to activate sterol receptor-binding protein-1c (SREBP-1c) independently of insulin, which, in turn, activates genes that are largely involved in DNL (Stanhope & Havel, 2008).

Insulin and glucose directly regulate lipid synthesis and secretion. Sterol receptor-binding protein-1c is a key transcription factor that is responsible for regulating fatty acid and cholesterol biosynthesis, and insulin controls its expression (Basciano et al., 2005). In all three major target insulin tissues of the body, namely liver, fat, and skeletal muscle, expression of SREBP-1c is enhanced by insulin. Similarly, under conditions of insulin resistance with resultant hyperinsulinemia, SREBP-1c is enhanced. Under conditions of insulin depletion, (namely through streptozotocin treatment), SREBP-1c is still expressed upon glucose, fructose or sucrose feeding. Together with the reduced insulin availability, it would have been reasonable to expect SREBP-1c downregulation, but such is not the case. With glucose feeding, a short-term peak of SREBP-1c is induced, with fructose being responsible for a gradual prolonged increase in SREBP-1c activity. The above proves that, independent of insulin signaling, carbohydrate, particularly fructose, availability can bring about lipogenesis (Basciano et al., 2005; Stanhope & Havel, 2008).

The mechanisms for fructose-induced IR share similarities with those that promote high-fat-induced IR. Neither fat nor fructose elicits insulin responses, and neither interferes with insulin signaling at common points in skeletal muscle. In hepatic cells, both high-fructose and high-fat diets elicit hepatic stress responses that activate inflammatory cascades (Lê & Tappy, 2006).

Intrahepatic VLDL production and secretion require the presence of available lipid substrate, which can be provided in unregulated amounts (acetyl-CoA and glycerol-3-phosphate) by entry of fructose into the liver (Stanhope & Havel, 2008). The assembly of triglyceride into VLDL is dependent upon apolipoprotein B100 (ApoB), which is considered highly atherosclerotic (Basciano et al., 2005; Havel 2005; Stanhope & Havel, 2008).

When the hepatic lipid concentration increases, the degradation of ApoB is dramatically reduced, and, under conditions of fructose consumption, ApoB concentrations may rise by as much as 25% (Basciano et al., 2005; Stanhope & Havel, 2008). Several short-term studies have shown fructose to promote unfavourable lipid profiles, with the hypertriglyceridemic effect being more pronounced in the longer term, together with increased postprandial levels of the atherogenic ApoB. Hypertriglyceridaemia is considered an independent risk factor for coronary heart disease, and even moderate increases in VLDL are associated with such changes as reduced HDL and small, dense LDL. The lipoprotein changes are strong components of the MS, and are recognised as risk factors for atherosclerotic disease (Havel, 2005).

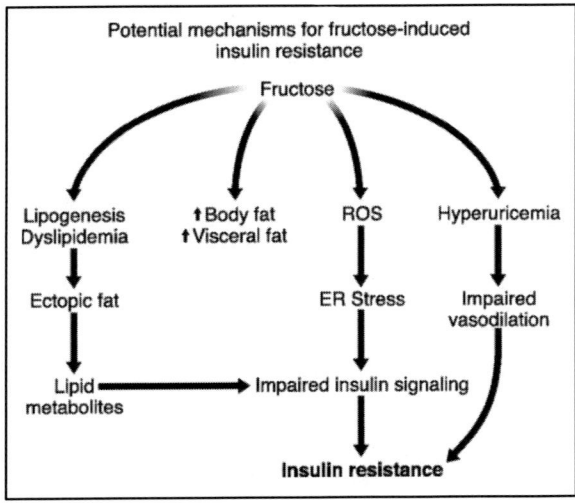

Source: Tappy & Lê, 2010.

Figure 10. The putative mechanisms that link fructose excess to MS.

Thus, the postprandial hypertriglyceridaemia seen after fructose ingestion is exacerbated in individuals with higher fasting insulin concentrations, suggesting a strong relationship between IR and the lipogenic effects of fructose (Elliott et al., 2002). Regardless of the mechanism, it is clear that fructose feeding can induce insulin resistance and glucose intolerance. Since the intake of fructose in the American diet has shown to have increased considerably over the past three decades, it is important to examine the effect of fructose on individuals who are predisposed to insulin resistance and glucose intolerance, such as those with PCOS.

Stanhope and Havel (2008) investigated the metabolic effects of beverages providing 25% of total calories of energy requirements for 10 weeks, in older, overweight men and women. In their interim report, both patient groups gained an average of 1.5 kg within 8 weeks. As measured by computerised tomography, the fructose group showed a significant increase in intra-abdominal fat, as opposed to the glucose group, who remained unchanged (Stanhope & Havel, 2008).

These researchers reported, based on interim results, that a high-fructose diet promotes the development of three of the cornerstone characteristics associated with MS, namely:

- dyslipidemia;
- insulin resistance; and
- increased visceral adiposity.

The evidence from various studies show that the regulation of appetite and gastro-intestinal hormones might be dysfunctional in subjects with PCOS (Bray et al., 2004; Elliott et al., 2002; Havel, 2005; Lê & Tappy, 2006; Moran et al., 2006; Teff et al., 2004). Both plasma insulin and leptin act in the central nervous system (CNS) in terms of the long-term regulation of energy homeostasis. Because fructose does not stimulate insulin, the consumption of foods and beverages with high-fructose content produces smaller postprandial insulin excursions than does consumption of glucose-containing carbohydrate. Leptin production is regulated by means of insulin responses to meals, with a time delay of several hours. A lower insulin response after ingestion of fructose would then be associated with lower serum leptin concentrations than would be the case after ingestion of glucose. Because of the anorexigenic effect of leptin, the lower levels of leptin after fructose intake would serve to enhance appetite and food intake. The combined effects of lowered circulating leptin and insulin in high-fructose diets could, therefore, increase the likelihood of hyperphagia, weight gain and its associated metabolic consequences (Bray et al., 2004; Elliott et al., 2002; Havel, 2005).

As in the study of PCOS and the adherence to diet/dropout rate, much attention has been given to the orexigenic gastric peptide, ghrelin, due to its potent effects on stimulating food intake in animals and humans. The researchers concerned showed that the relative elevation of ghrelin after fructose ingestion suggests the failure of fructose to suppress ghrelin, along with reduced insulin and leptin, which could contribute to decreased satiety and to increased food intake during long-term fructose consumption. Glucose-mediated insulin stimulation elevates circulating levels of leptin, and, in turn, the orexigenic gastric peptide, ghrelin, is suppressed (Teff et al., 2004).

2.9. THE ROLE OF ANTI-MÜLLERIAN HORMONE

In studies on both adult women and adolescents, anti-Müllerian hormone (AMH) has been suggested as a diagnostic tool for PCOS (Arora, 2017; Rencber et al., 2018). AMH is a glycol-protein mainly produced in the pre-antral and small antral follicles, the same place as the origin of hyperandrogenism in PCOS. The anti-Müllerian hormone plays an important role in recruitment of primordial ovarian follicles, as well as selection of the dominant follicle (Rencber et al., 2018). Since no clear cut-off values are yet available for AMH, it has not been included in any diagnostic criteria for PCOS (Reinehr et al., 2017).

According to Arora (2017), the level of AMH is increased in women with PCOS, which could be related to levels of LH, insulin, and androgens. Genetic factors might also contribute to over-expression of AMH. Since individual granulosa cells produce AMH, the increased number of antral follicles in PCOS would suggest a higher number of granulosa cells, and a higher formation of AMH (Arora, 2017; Rencber et al., 2018). A study has shown that, per granulosa cell, there might be a 75-fold increase in AMH production in females with PCOS, as opposed to non-PCOS women (Arora, 2017).

Both FSH and AMH are regarded as markers of functional ovarian reserve, reflecting different stages of follicular development. Anti-Müllerian hormone would be an accurate marker of early ovarian antral follicle number, while FSH would mostly represent follicular maturation in the last two weeks, in the time when follicles become susceptible to menstrual hormones (Reinehr et al., 2017). Anti-Müllerian hormone plays an inhibitory role in follicular recruitment and development, and elevated levels of AMH contribute to early follicular arrest. FSH-regulated aromatase production is also inhibited by AMH, leading to hyperandrogenism, and further exacerbating the effect of insulin. The possibility of a paracrine effect on the theca cells, suggests theca cell dysregulation, and excessive androgen production (Arora, 2017).

Increased serum levels of AMH could be predictive of the success of interventions such as diet and exercise, ovulation induction and ovarian drilling, while improvement in several parameters following treatment, leads to a decline in serum levels of AMH. Reinehr et al. (2017) conducted a longitudinal study of obese girls, with and without PCOS, in a one-year lifestyle intervention. The study concluded that elevated AMH was predictive of poor response to different interventions, including weight loss. This supports a possible role for AMH in the pathophysiology of PCOS (Arora, 2017; Reinehr et al., 2017).

A study published in 2012, reported that AMH is an accurate measure for diagnosis of PCOS in adults, when it replaces ultrasonic evidence of polycystic ovaries (Agapova et al., 2014).

2.10. GENETIC AND ANDROGEN EXPOSURE FACTORS AND PCOS

Studies have shown an approximate 70% concordance of PCOS in mono-zygotic twins, which suggests that PCOS is a highly hereditary condition. The male and female first-degree relatives of PCOS women, show metabolic and reproductive abnormalities, including insulin resistance, type-2 diabetes mellitus and lipid abnormalities in both males and females, and oligomenorrhea polycystic ovaries and androgen excess in the females (Arora, 2017; Penaforte et al., 2009). The variability of the phenotypic features in different families and within the same family, emphasises the substantial contribution of environmental factors, especially obesity, in the manifestation of PCOS (Penaforte et al., 2009).

Glucose-stimulated hyperinsulinemia develops as early as four years of age (4 yrs), and continues throughout puberty in girls from such heredity. During assessment of β-cell function in pre-pubertal girls from ages eight to fourteen (8-14 yrs), using fasting indices of insulin resistance and insulin responses during administration of an intravenous glucose tolerance test, insulin resistance and β-cell dysfunction were shown. Follow-up of peri-pubertal girls with PCOS mothers, showed that the β-cell dysfunction persisted for over two years, suggesting a hereditary abnormality in pancreatic β-cell function. Several epigenetic factors and signaling molecules have been studied in this regard (Macut et al., 2017). Studies on gene expression of different tissues have identified pathways for the pathophysiology of PCOS, and might be different between lean and obese PCOS women (Arora, 2017).

Exposure to androgen excess during fetal development, as a result of hyperandrogenemia from the mother, may lead to features of PCOS and/or metabolic syndrome, which might only start to present at puberty or even sooner (Macut et al., 2017). Should the fetus be exposed to high levels of androgens, the development of programming of a normal HPO-axis could be severely compromised, resulting in excessive secretion of LH, the development of insulin resistance, and resulting anovulation. In addition, prenatal overexposure to androgens affects the developing female offspring permanently, inducing an increase in β-cell number. This alters the primary response of the pancreas to glucose, implying future derangements in glucose response and metabolism (Macut et al., 2017).

2.11. Environmental Factors and PCOS

An array of environmental factors could also have an impact on the pathophysiology of PCOS. These factors include pollutants, psychological stress, social environment, as well as belief-systems, carried over through generations. This may also include factors which unknowingly favour the development of PCOS, such as ethnic and traditional beliefs about eating habits and other factors of lifestyle.

2.11.1. Smoking

Although the mechanism is not defined, smoking negatively influences the fertility of female smokers. The negative consequences of chronic smoking include rapid depletion of ovarian follicular reserve, delayed conception, increased risk of miscarriage in both natural and assisted pregnancies, and increased risk of birth defects (Silvestris et al., 2018).

2.11.2. Drugs, Caffeine and Alcohol

A number of over-the-counter, easily accessible drugs that might be taken daily or occasionally, are known to impact on fertility. Non-steroidal anti-inflammatory drugs (NSAIDs), frequently used for the treatment of pain or inflammation, are *defined ovulation inhibitors*. Cytotoxic chemotherapy as anti-cancer treatment also causes ovarian failure in women.

High intakes of caffeine (above 400mg per day, which equals 4 cups of brewed coffee, 10 tins of cola drink or two "energy" drinks (Mayo Clinic, 2018)) are associated with an increased risk of pregnancy loss.

In alcohol abuse, the alterations to liver metabolism and neuro-psychological damage act synergistically with stress factors to prevent oocyte maturation (Silvestris et al., 2018).

2.11.3. Physical Activity

The advantages of regular physical activity, such as decreasing abdominal fat, glucose levels, blood lipids, insulin resistance, as well as improved menstrual cyclicity, lowered testosterone levels, and increased SHBG, favour ovulation and fertility. To the contrary, excessive physical activity could be closely linked to negative effects on the whole body, including the reproductive system. Intense agonistic (highly-competitive) sports, may produce the syndrome known as "female athlete triad", characterized by amenorrhea, osteoporosis and eating disorder, as per definition by the American College of Sports Medicine (Silvestris et al., 2018).

2.11.4. Environmental Pollutants

Several investigative studies by the US Occupational Safety and Health Administration (2016) have shown that chronic exposure to specific chemicals are associated with reduced fertility and the tendency towards recurrent miscarriage.

2.11.4.1. Organic Solvents

This is a common class of compounds used frequently and routinely in commercial industries. They were discovered in the late 19th century from the coal-tar industry. Their use grew wide and diverse in both developed and developing countries. However, only in the 1920s, the introduction of chlorinated solvents led to reports of toxicity. There are thousands of different organic solvents, but only a few have been tested for neurotoxicity. Industrial workers may experience occupational exposure, but other individuals may be exposed environmentally through contaminated water, soil, food or air. Exposure often involves a mixture of solvents and the most common examples are paints and glues. Absorption of organic solvents may take place through inhalation, dermal contact, or ingestion (Rutchik, 2014).

2.11.4.2. Aromatic Amines

Aromatic amines are chemical substances widely used as precursor to pesticides, pharmaceuticals, and dyes. They are also used for all coloured textiles, dyed, printed and coated. Aromatic amines also abound in hair dyes, fluorescent dyes and certain drugs, as listed in Table 5 (Vogt & Gerulis, 2005).

Table 5. Names and examples of aromatic amines

Representative aromatic amines		
Aromatic ring	**Name of parent amines**	**Example**
acridine	aminoacridines	fluorescent dyes
benzene	aniline	substituted anilines
benzene	phenylenediamines	the antioxidant p-phenylenediamine
naphthalene	naphthylamines	the dye Methyl violet
purine	aminopurines	the nucleobase guanine
pyridine	aminopyridines	the drug tenoxicam
pyrimidine	aminopyrimidines	the nucleobase cytosine
quinoline	aminoquinolines	the drug primaquine
toluene	toluidines	the pharmaceutical prilocain
toluene	diaminotoluenes	the hair dye ingredient 2,5-diaminotoluene

Source: Vogt & Gerulius, 2005.

2.11.4.3. Heavy Metals

Heavy metals could be defined as minerals that are 5 000 times heavier than the gravity of water. They build up over time, and contaminate our bodies, as well as the environment. Heavy metals include lead, mercury, arsenic, cadmium, nickel and others. Aluminium is not considered a heavy metal, but it behaves like one. Cadmium specifically, causes atherosclerosis and calcification of the body organs and blood vessels, and compromises all functions.

Heavy metals have been identified as a factor which could impact on the reproductive system, and cause infertility through accelerating the aging process and prematurely depleting ovarian follicular reserves. They also accelerate the inflammatory process and prevent the effective elimination of toxic substances.

High levels of mercury may interfere with both male and female fertility. Through accumulation in the brain and nervous system, they damage neurotransmitters and affect the HPO-axis through suppressing gonadotropins (FSH and LH).

Accumulation of heavy metals in the ovaries disrupts the production of estrogen and progesterone and cause defective oocyte development. Other fertility problems due to heavy metals include long or short menstrual cycles, recurrent loss of pregnancy or miscarriage, unexplained infertility, PCOS, and sperm abnormalities. Tips for prevention include:

- Removal of dental amalgams;
- Avoiding seafood;
- Avoiding exposure to all paints and glues;
- Stop smoking and avoiding being present in tobacco smoke (Gerhard et al., 1998).

2.11.5. Shift Work

Insulin resistance, which is considered the cornerstone in the development of PCOS, may also be the result of lifestyle factors such as shift work (especially night shifts), insufficient sleep and lack of physical activity. There have been reports that nurses in particular, working night shifts, are at risk of developing insulin resistance. Shift work can also lead to sleep deprivation and lack of exercise. The relevance of shift work to the pathophysiology of PCOS is difficult to interpret, since long and short menstrual cycles may result from shift work (Lim et al., 2016).

A study carried out in by Lim et al. (2016) in Singapore between 2011 and 2015, on healthy women, aged 21 to 45 years, showed that shift work, short sleep duration and lack of exercise were not linked with any ovarian or androgenic measures that might define PCOS. Short sleep duration, rather than shift work, showed significant association with menstrual cycle length. Women having fewer than 6 hours' sleep, showed a 3.9-fold increased risk of short menstrual cycles, of less than 25 days, and a 1.7-fold increased risk for long menstrual cycles of more than 35 days (Lim et al., 2016).

Recent findings also suggest that women with diagnosed PCOS experience disturbances in both circadian rhythm and sleep. The disruption of pulsatile FSH and LH secretion associated with disordered sleep, may disturb the luteinisation of granulosa cells, resulting in a defective luteal phase, and shorter menstrual cycles. However, no association was found between short sleep duration and changes in reproductive hormone levels in the Lim et al. (2016) study. Their findings were consistent with those of other studies, that short sleep duration is significantly associated with metabolic dysfunctions, including higher BMI, elevated fasting insulin levels and higher risk of insulin resistance. Women who slept longer than 6 hours, had a reduced risk of IR over those who slept for less than 6 hours.

The results suggest that women who get insufficient sleep are at risk of IR and menstrual irregularities. Sleep may be an important protector against ovulatory dysfunction, fertility problems, and IR (Lim et al., 2016).

2.12. THE ROLE OF APPETITE REGULATION IN PCOS

The sustainability of weight reduction diets in obese women with PCOS is well known to be poor over the long term, with little maintenance of weight loss. Huber-Buchholz, Carey and Norman (1999) and Moran et al. (2006) substantiated this view by referring to the 26% to 38% dropout rate for PCOS sufferers on weight-loss regimes, as opposed to 8% to 9% in non-PCOS subjects. In an experimental co-hort study by Weidemann (2012), where 86 overweight and obese females with PCOS were studied, the dropout rate after the first dietary consultation was 50%, with a further dropout of 41% between the first and second follow-up visits.

Although anecdotal reports of increased difficulty with weight loss in PCOS abound, the phenomenon has never been scientifically proven. The high dropout rate among PCOS sufferers might be due to abnormal appetite regulation, leading to difficulty with energy restriction. This implies that PCOS women comprise a population that requires intensive long-term dietary coaching, with regular follow-up and support. Dietary strategies to maximise satiety are certainly applicable to help the patients achieve and maintain a desirable body weight (Moran et al., 2006). However, there is some evidence that derangements in appetite control hormones exist in patients with PCOS, and that this may account for deregulated hunger and satiety cues (Farshchi et al., 2007; Marsh & Brand-Miller, 2005, Moran et al., 2006, Moran & Norman, 2004). Satiety after eating a meal (postprandial satiety), has been found to be less, and hunger after eating a meal (postprandial hunger) is more, before and after weight loss, in PCOS women as opposed to weight-matched controls (Moran et al., 2007).

The hormones that have most frequently been studied for their involvement in appetite regulation in PCOS, are cholecystokinin (CCK), ghrelin and leptin.

Hunger and appetite are regulated in the hypothalamus through a cluster of neurons (nerve cells), referred to as the arcuate nucleus. An intricate dynamic exists between neurons that receive satiety cues and those that receive hunger cues. It appears that insulin resistance starts in the hypothalamus through inflammation, leading to attenuated signaling for hunger and satiety (Sears & Perry, 2015).

Interestingly, the only hormone of those connected to appetite regulation that stimulates appetite, also referred to as orexigenic, is ghrelin. The other hormones such as leptin, and CCK, act to suppress hunger, also referred to as anorexigenic (Moran et al., 2006; Moran et al., 2007). The question still remains whether these abnormalities of appetite regulation might be implicated in the pathogenesis of PCOS, or whether PCOS brings about appetite deregulation.

2.12.1. Cholecystokinin

The hormone cholecystokinin (CCK) is released in the duodenum in response to postprandial protein and fat, and acts by delaying gastric emptying, thereby increasing satiety and reducing meal size and caloric intake, and assisting with meal termination. Compared with weight-matched controls, there is a reduced postprandial CCK response in overweight women with PCOS, which suggests dysregulation of appetite control by CCK in PCOS (Moran et al., 2006; Moran et al., 2007).

This short-acting hormone works to suppress hunger by directly interacting with the hypothalamus via the vagus nerve. In animal models being fed a diet high in saturated fat with a view to create insulin resistance through inflammation in the hypothalamus, the satiety signals by CCK were attenuated (Sears & Perry, 2015).

2.12.2. Ghrelin

Ghrelin is an orexigenic hormone that is produced primarily by the endocrine cells in the fundus of the stomach, and is the only gastro-intestinal hormone in humans, that has been found to stimulate appetite (Farshchi et al., 2007; Moran et al., 2004; Moran et al., 2006; Moran et al., 2007). The most important function of ghrelin, is stimulation of food intake and long-term regulation of body weight and energy balance. Levels of ghrelin increase sharply in anticipation of a meal, and again decrease 2 to 3 hours after the meal. The sharp increase stimulates hunger through action on the hypothalamic arcuate nucleus and produces satiety after a meal, through reduced production and thus decreased levels of ghrelin. In obese subjects with or without PCOS, fasting levels of ghrelin are decreased, so that postprandial suppression of ghrelin is smaller, causing diminished satiety after meals and compromised meal termination. Although the down-regulation of ghrelin in obesity might be improved by weight loss and fasting levels of ghrelin improved, the restoration of ghrelin homeostasis seems to be impaired in PCOS. A study of 26 women with PCOS were compared to 61 healthy controls. Serum levels of ghrelin in the PCOS group were found to be significantly lower than in the control group (even matching the ghrelin levels found in gastrectomised women), and strongly relating to the degree of IR (Schöfl et al., 2002).

Apart from appetite control, ghrelin also has a variety of other functions, such as glucose metabolism and control, increased inflammation and vasodilatation, and ovarian function. Ghrelin receptors are found on ovarian tissue, which suggests a possible reproductive influence by ghrelin. The lower fasting ghrelin levels seen in PCOS subjects might also be a reflection of the increased metabolic, diabetic and reproductive dysfunction characteristic to the condition, rather than abnormality in appetite regulation (Moran et al., 2007).

The amount of weight loss that is required to bring about ghrelin restoration is also unknown. The impaired satiety through down regulation of fasting ghrelin and impaired postprandial ghrelin suppression might explain the difficulty in adhering to weight-loss regimes that seems to be experienced amongst PCOS women. Therefore, long-term weight loss regimes should be based on strategies to improve satiety. Regular follow-up and support are considered crucial in the weight management of overweight or obese subjects with PCOS (Moran et al., 2006).

It seems that treatment with Metformin, in the case of insulin resistant PCOS, increases serum ghrelin levels. This is suggestive of a link between insulin sensitivity and ghrelin, indicating that the deregulated ghrelin response in PCOS with IR, could be normalized with Metformin therapy. Although restoration of the ghrelin response would lead to improved postprandial ghrelin suppression and improved meal termination, ghrelin levels do not correlate with BMI. There is a much stronger correlation between ghrelin, insulin resistance and carbohydrate metabolism, probably because ghrelin is also expressed in pancreatic β-cells, hence it may directly inhibit insulin release (Schöfl et al., 2002).

2.12.3. Leptin

The biology of leptin was uncovered through research on leptin deficiency and studying the effects of leptin repletion in both animals and humans. In humans, leptin deficient states include only genetic leptin deficiency, which is extremely rare, starvation situations (anorexia nervosa), and untreated insulin deficiency. These states are associated with increased appetite, decreased energy expenditure and neuro-endocrine dysfunction, as well as hyperglycemia in the untreated insulin-deficient subjects. Administration of exogenous leptin reduced the appetite, corrected the hyperglycemia and reversed endocrine dysfunction.

Leptin is an anorexigenic hormone which is produced by the fat cells, and plays a key role in regulation of energy intake and expenditure, including appetite and metabolism. It is probably the most important fat-derived hormone, and elevated levels are strongly associated with BMI, insulin effectivity and glucose metabolism. Since leptin is derived from body fat, an increase in fat cells results in an increase in leptin production. Leptin has been shown to be a potential regulator for many reproductive functions, such as folliculogenesis, ovarian production of steroid hormones, development of dominant follicles, endometrial development, and functions relating to lactation. A deficiency of leptin has been linked to both infertility and delayed puberty in humans and rodents. Leptin is now considered as a possible link between nutrition and reproduction (Nomair et al., 2014).

Ovarian granulosa and theca cells contain abundant leptin receptors, and when these cells were treated with leptin, production of steroid hormones was significantly reduced. Leptin also has a beneficial effect on the HPO-axis level, serving as a trigger to puberty and reproductive development, both in males and females (Nomair et al., 2014). Leptin supports reproductive competence through many aspects, and leptin dysregulation has been implicated in the development of PCOS and other anovulatory conditions (Myers et al., 2012; Nomair et al., 2014).

Obesity has been found to be associated with elevated levels of leptin, and in literature, overweight females with PCOS, both with and without IR, have shown higher leptin levels than their non-PCOS counterparts (Nomair et al., 2014). In obesity, leptin levels are much elevated in comparison to lean individuals, but the elevated leptin fails to reduce excess body weight to normal. The poor efficacy of endogenous leptin has given rise to the notion of "leptin resistance", implicating that leptin action is impaired, which facilitates the progression of obesity and limits the potential action of treatment with exogenous leptin (Myers et al., 2012). Nomair et al. (2014)

concluded that the CNS receptors, which are normally very sensitive towards leptin levels, are protected from high leptin (hyperleptinemia) levels by a saturatable transport system over the blood-brain barrier. Thus, peripheral leptin receptors, in contrast, are exposed to high leptin concentrations, which have possible negative effects on the reproductive system.

Nomair et al. (2014) also concluded that leptin has a dual effect on reproduction, and that the site of action differs according to the levels of circulating leptin.

Chapter 3

BRIEF OVERVIEW OF DRUGS AND SURGERY USED FOR TREATMENT IN PCOS

The consensus groups discussed thus far, regarding the diagnosis of PCOS, together with opinion leaders in the field of PCOS, agree that change of lifestyle and improvements in dietary practices should form the first line of therapy in the treatment of PCOS (Macut et al., 2017; Penaforte et al., 2009; Rotterdam, 2003; Saleem & Rizvi, 2017; Thessaloniki workshop group, 2008). However, certain drug treatments and surgical procedures are used as treatment of this condition both for alleviating debilitating symptoms and assisting in fertilization, before turning to assisted reproductive technology (ART).

Several international guidelines from different groups exist for use of drugs and surgical interventions for ovulation induction, such as those of the National Institute of Clinical Excellence (NICE) guidelines published in 2004, and the Society of Obstetricians and Gynecologists of Canada (SOGC) published in 2010 (Saha, Kaur & Saha, 2012). A recent publication suggested that lifestyle improvements, pharmacological therapy and bariatric surgery become the main interventions for management of obese PCOS and preventing metabolic co-morbidities, and that lifestyle interventions resulting in weight loss only, is sometimes insufficient for treating PCOS in females with normal BMI (Saleem & Rizvi, 2017).

With PCOS commonly associated with hyperinsulinemia, insulin resistance, and obesity, these patients are at a high risk for developing T2DM and metabolic syndrome. The rate at which normal glucose tolerance can progress to impaired glucose tolerance and T2DM can be as high as 5% to 15% in three years, substantially increasing the risk of acute myocardial infarction and stroke in obese women with PCOS. Obesity and PCOS have many common features linked to insulin resistance, and all three modalities of treatment (lifestyle modification, drug treatment and surgical intervention) have their place in optimal treatment of PCOS (Saleem & Rizvi, 2017).

Although lifestyle management and improvement remains the key metabolic strategy for PCOS, there is still no clear recommendation to the diet for PCOS women. It seems that even a moderate and short-lasting reduction in carbohydrate of any kind, could reduce fasting insulin, which in turn would be followed by amelioration of insulin sensitivity. (Macut et al., 2017).

As much as it is postulated that the combination of diet and exercise could ameliorate the metabolic, hormonal and reproductive indices of women with PCOS, as with the dietary regimens, no established programmes of physical training for PCOS women have yet seen the light. The inclusion of exercise is also a field of specialization, which should be approached with an educated and experienced trainer, regarding the special needs and hormonal environment of the female with PCOS.

3.1. MENSTRUAL IRREGULARITIES AND THE USE OF ORAL CONTRACEPTIVE PILLS

The number of menstrual cycles carries less importance than prevention of endometrial hyperplasia. The induction of menstruation, most commonly through the use of oral contraceptive pills (OCPs), either cyclically or continuously, prevents hyperproliferation of the uterus. Treatment with combined OCPs (estrogen with a progestogen) is a first-line treatment for

PCOS in women not seeking pregnancy, and is supported by guidelines. OCPs assists in regulation of the menstrual cycle, and reduce androgen production and its corresponding features, such as hirsutism and acne (Barthelmess & Naz, 2014; Saha et al., 2012; Saleem & Rizvi, 2017).

Estrogen assists in elevating SHBG levels, and reducing LH and FSH levels, which in turn suppress testosterone levels and ovarian androgen production. Recent studies support a new treatment option, which include insulin sensitizers such as Metformin, anti-androgens, or both, with potential beneficial effects on metabolic abnormalities. This treatment option is particularly useful in treatment of adolescents with PCOS (Barthelmess & Naz, 2014; Saha et al., 2012). No long-term studies have been done on the metabolic risks of taking OCPs, and since an increased risk of cardio-metabolic effects have been shown among the general population, women with PCOS should have an even greater risk. This area of research is currently extremely relevant, since OCPs have been used as the primary treatment of PCOS for decades (Barthelmess & Naz, 2014).

3.2. Fertility

3.2.1. Anti-Estrogens

Clomiphene citrate (CC) is an oral medication that can be used to stimulate ovulation through blocking estrogen receptors at the hypothalamus. When this happens, the hypothalamus is stimulated to release follicle stimulating hormone (FSH), and luteinizing hormone (LH), prompting a normal menstrual cycle. This is normally a first line of treatment for 12 months, because of the likelihood of stimulating ovulation. Women treated with CC should be informed of the likelihood of multiple pregnancies (Barthelmess & Naz, 2014; Saha et al., 2012; Thessaloniki workshop group, 2008). Treatment with CC has shown high conception rates in thin women with ovulatory dysfunction, but the possibility of a multiple pregnancy remains a major drawback (Saha et al., 2012).

3.2.2. Insulin Sensitizers

The most commonly-used insulin sensitizer, Metformin, is a drug used in the maintenance of type-2 diabetes mellitus (T2DM). Together with controlled dietary intake and increased physical activity, Metformin works to control the blood sugar level by controlling gluconeogenesis in the liver (Gluconeogenesis comprises the formation of glucose by the liver, using the "backbones" of fat and amino acids, rather than carbohydrates). Like OCPs, Metformin has been used in the treatment of PCOS for decades, and research has confirmed its usefulness in treating hyperinsulinemia and insulin resistance. It has also been shown to reduce androgen production and help control the menstrual cycle in women with PCOS (Barthelmess & Naz, 2014).

In women with PCOS, Metformin helps to lower fasting insulin, but does not assist with lowering BMI. Of particular note may be the fact that Metformin has no superiority over weight loss, with regards to improvement in ovulation frequency. Also, it seems that the only advantage to adding Metformin to CC treatment, lies with women who have a BMI greater than 35kg/m^2 (Thessaloniki workshop group, 2008). Women prescribed Metformin should be clearly informed about its side-effects, which could include gastro-intestinal disturbances such as nausea, vomiting and diarrhea (Saha et al., 2012).

3.2.3. Ovarian Drilling

Laparoscopic ovarian drilling is a surgical treatment that can trigger ovulation in women who have PCOS. Electrocautery or a laser is used to destroy parts of the ovaries. This surgical intervention is not associated with multiple pregnancies, and should be offered to women who have not responded to treatment with CC (Saha et al., 2012).

3.2.4. Gonadotropins

Guidelines from the different governing bodies for fertility treatment should be followed by specialists, when gonadotropins are used for ovulation induction, and should be seen as a second-line therapy. Close monitoring through ultrasound and laboratory work are required. The drawbacks of this line of therapy are the high cost, risk of multiple pregnancy, and risk of ovarian hyperstimulation syndrome (OHSS) (Barthelmess & Naz, 2014; Saha et al., 2012).

3.2.5. Assisted Reproductive Technology

There are several procedures for assisted reproductive technology (ART), such as artificial insemination (AI) and/or in vitro fertilization (IVF). Artificial insemination involves the delivering of sperm directly into the cervix or uterus of the female, while IVF refers to the harvesting of mature follicles or oocytes from the female and fertilizing them with sperm in a laboratory. The fertilized egg or eggs are then implanted into the uterus. One cycle of IVF takes about two weeks, and IVF is considered the most effective form of ART (Mayo Clinic, 2018).

The first step in any form of ART is hyperstimulation of the ovaries with a view of producing multiple follicles. This is done by using gonadotropins, but some women have a severe response to this, leading to ovarian hyperstimulation syndrome (OHSS) (Barthelmess & Naz, 2014). Successful ART is largely dependent on a harvest of follicles or oocytes of high quality. It is imperative that the female is given at least 16 weeks to implement lifestyle changes for improved ovarian function and ovulation, and pre-treatment weight loss, with or without concurrent contraceptive therapy (Saleem & Rizvi, 2018), not disregarding the fact that during this time, her chances of spontaneous pregnancy are elevated by roughly 50% (unpublished data, Weidemann, 2012).

3.2.6. Bariatric Surgery

This extreme form of surgery is only recommended in morbidly obese women with PCOS, where co-morbidities such as cardiovascular disease and diabetes are present. One year after a bariatric procedure, these women have shown significant improvements in cardio-metabolic disease, and decreases in BMI, HbA1c, total cholesterol, LDL, and triglyceride levels (Saleem & Rizvi, 2017).

A comprehensive overview of the benefits and detriments of bariatric surgery for obese females with PCOS falls beyond the scope of this book.

Chapter 4

ALTERNATIVE AND COMPLEMENTARY TREATMENTS FOR USE IN PCOS

Although using some alternative and complementary supplements has been beneficial in the treatment of PCOS, it remains imperative that the treating physician is made aware of what is being taken, as well as the dosage.

4.1. MYO-INOSITOL AND D-CHIRO-INOSITOL

Overweight women with PCOS respond well to insulin-sensitizers, such as Metformin, which help to reduce serum androgens, and restore ovulation. However, several limitations have been linked to their use: Metformin induces symptoms of the gastro-intestinal tract, such as bloating, diarrhea and nausea. Other insulin-sensitizing agents, such as troglitazone (TZD), have other practical limitations, such as induction of weight gain, and more recently, the association with increased coronary artery disease and myocardial infarction (Nordio & Proietti, 2012).

Myo-inositol (MI) and D-chiro-inositol (DCI) might be the most researched alternative nutritional supplements for use in PCOS (Grassi, 2013). Inositol is a six-carbon polyol which belongs both to the sugar family and the B-vitamins, being called a vitamin-like sugar. It occurs naturally in the tissues of humans and animals, and has many forms (isomers) of which MI and DCI are the most abundant. Both MI and DCI are incorporated into inositolphosphoglycans (IPGs), acting as second messengers to insulin, and some of the actions of insulin are facilitated by these IPGs. Since PCOS is linked to insulin resistance, any defect in tissue availability or deranged metabolism of the inositols or IPGs second messenger pathway, might exacerbate insulin resistance (Grassi, 2013; Saleem & Rizvi, 2017). Both MI and DCI have shown favourable results in improving the aspects of PCOS, such as insulin sensitivity, ovulation and oocyte quality, improved levels of androgens and improving inflammation, hypertension, dyslipidemia and weight loss. These benefits make MI and DCI important supplements that should be considered as a part of the first-line of treatment for PCOS (Grassi, 2013; Nordio & Proietti, 2012).

Inositols are known for their part in enzyme activation that plays a pivotal role in glucose metabolism. MI is the precursor of inositolphophoglycan (IPG) mediators that support glucose metabolism. Studies suggest that a tissue deficiency of MI or an altered metabolism of IPG mediators, may contribute to insulin resistance (Nordio & Proietti, 2012; Saleem & Rizvi 2017).

Myo-inositol has been found to be more beneficial at improving the metabolic profile, while DCI has a better effect on reducing androgens than MI. With Inositol supplementation, spontaneous ovulation might be restored, leading to improved fertility in women with PCOS (Saleem & Rizvi, 2017).

However, when DCI is given alone at high dose, there is an unfavourable effect on oocyte quality. Furthermore, research has shown that when MI and DCI are given at a physiological ratio of 40:1, clinical results improve favourably. The optimal ratio of MI: DCI varies in each body tissue, according to its needs. The dosage to achieve maximum effectivity of combined MI with DCI in combination for treatment of overweight PCOS patients, who need to control insulin and minimize risk of developing MS, and in a ratio of 40:1, is 2g to 4g per day. Unlike other insulin-sensitizing agents, no side effects have been reported after MI and DCI administration (Nordio & Proietti, 2012; Saleem & Rizvi, 2017).

4.2. BERBERINE

Berberine is a type of isoquinoline-derivative alkaloid which is extracted from several Chinese medicinal herbs, amongst others Copitidis Rhizome (Huanglian), Cortex Phellodendri (Huangbai), and Hydrastis Canadensis (goldenseal) (Wei et al., 2012). In China, berberine has been used for the treatment of diarrhea, and has been found to have glucose-lowering effects. It is also believed to increase the success rate of IVF, following the beneficial effect on insulin resistance. Berberine given at a dosage of 0.5g three times a day, showed improvement in insulin resistance in 120 women with PCOS. Three months of berberine treatment prior to an IVF cycle also increased live birth rate in a prospective study of 150 women (Li et al., 2015).

The first study to evaluate the effect of berberine treatment alone on menstrual pattern, ovulation rate, and hormonal and metabolic profiles in anovulatory women suffering from PCOS, was done by Li et al. and published in 2015. In other studies, fasting glucose was shown to be reduced with dosages of 0.3g to 0.5g of berberine three times daily, while the administration of 0.5g three times per day for three months showed improvements in plasma glucose, triglycerides, total cholesterol and LDL levels, compared to placebo. The researchers also found that the use of berberine alone could improve ovulation rate in their study, similar to that of Metformin alone in other studies, but concluded that further studies are needed to compare the efficacy in ovulation induction between berberine, metformin, CC, or a combination.

Wei et al. (2012) reported that, as a main constituent of Chinese medicine, berberine shows promising potential in the prevention and treatment of metabolic disorders, including weight control, reduction in cholesterol, anti-lipogenic and hypoglycaemic effects. Several trials have reported the ability of berberine to reduce body weight (as well as the ratio of white adipose tissue to body weight), but also to increase energy expenditure and the consumption of lipid metabolites as the primary fuel source in obese animals (An et al., 2014; Wei et al., 2012).

There has been little research on the effect of berberine on reproductive hormones. In a recent study where insulin resistance was induced on theca cells, berberine effectively antagonized excessive testosterone production. The mechanism of berberine-reducing hyperandrogenism remains unclear, but it may be related to the remarkable effect of berberine on the amelioration of IR (Wei et al., 2012).

The length of time needed for either berberine or Metformin to exert their metabolic effects in PCOS females undergoing gonadotropin ovarian stimulation, is not yet defined, and treatment is normally stopped on the day of downregulation. The study by An et al. (2014) was designed to validate the effect of berberine or metformin pre-treatment, based on the hypothesis that normalising the endocrine changes in PCOS women during the *85 days* necessary for primordial cells to reach pre-ovulatory status, would facilitate the IVF process, thus choosing 12 weeks of pre-treatment. They found that both berberine and Metformin achieved a significant improvement in pregnancy rates with a much lower risk of OHSS in women undergoing IVF. More research is needed to determine whether berberine treatment could be continued during the pregnancy, like Metformin, with greater beneficial effects (An et al., 2014).

No toxic effects of berberine have been demonstrated at the doses used in clinical situations (0.5g three times daily), and no marked changes in renal or hepatic function were observed. Wei et al. (2012) concluded that, in comparison to Metformin, berberine showed similar metabolic effects on improved insulin sensitivity and reduction of hyperandrogenemia. Berberine appeared to have a better effect on changes in body composition and dyslipidemia. The underlying mechanisms of action of berberine needs to be clarified in longer term studies in women with PCOS.

4.3. N-Acetyl Cysteine

Clomiphene resistance is defined as the failure to ovulate after receiving 150mg of CC per days for 5 days per cycle, for a minimum of 3 cycles. CC resistance is quite common and occurs in 15% to 40% of women with PCOS. Obesity, insulin resistance and hyperandrogenemia are the main factors that contribute to CC resistance (Saha, Kaur & Saha, 2013).

N-acetyl cysteine (NAC) is the acylated variant of the amino acid L-cysteine. NAC is converted in vivo into metabolites that promote detoxification through potent stimulation of the body's main anti-oxidant glutathione, which acts directly as a free-radical scavenger. Historically, NAC has been used as a mucolytic in respiratory conditions, but it has apparent benefit in many other conditions such as human immunodeficiency virus (HIV) infection, heavy-metal poisoning, epilepsy, and acetaminophen poisoning. In the human body, NAC is primarily a powerful anti-oxidant, but also acts on insulin secretion from pancreatic cells and insulin receptors on erythrocytes (red blood cells). It has anti-apoptotic effects, preserves vascular integrity and due to its strong anti-oxidant properties, NAC plays a role in immunological functions (Saha et al., 2013).

The possible beneficial effects of NAC on ovulation in CC-resistant PCOS, has been discussed in the literature. Some researchers have noted that the combination of CC and NAC improves ovulation and pregnancy rates in these women. A study in 2007 reported that the addition of NAC to a CC regimen in PCOS increases ovulation rates significantly (Saha et al., 2013).

Grassi (2013) reported on a study in 2011, in which the effects of NAC and Metformin were compared. One hundred women with PCOS were divided to receive either 500mg Metformin three times daily, or 600mg NAC three times daily for 24 weeks. Equal and significant improvements were seen in both treatment groups regarding BMI, hirsutism, fasting insulin, free testosterone and menstrual irregularity. NAC proved superior to Metformin in improvements in the lipid-profile.. The women taking NAC also had significant improvements in testosterone, cholesterol and triglyceride levels.

Studies have concluded that NAC not only improves the lipid profile, hormone levels and ovulation, but also the long-term health status of women with PCOS through improvement of oxidative stress and insulin sensitivity. Since NAC has no adverse effects, it may be regarded as an appropriate substitute for insulin-sensitizing medications in treating PCOS (Saha et al., 2012).

4.4. Resveratrol

Resveratrol, a natural polyphenolic compound (3,5,4-tritri-hydroxystilbene) is naturally found in the skins of grapes, red wine, peanuts and peanut butter, berries, celery and several medicinal plants. Resveratrol has been found to have anti-oxidant and anti-inflammatory properties, and depending on the cell type, it can act as both a pro-apoptotic and anti-apoptotic agent. In animal studies, resveratrol can significantly increase the number of oocytes, decrease the atretic follicles, and inhibit apoptosis during the primordial-to-developing-follicle transition. A study in rodents showed that resveratrol protected oocytes from induced cytotoxicity because the resveratrol facilitated the decrease of free radicals. Unfortunately, information of the beneficial effects of resveratrol on reproductive functions of the ovary is lacking (Rencber et al., 2018).

The main beneficial effects of resveratrol are contributed to its activation of silent information regulator-1 (SIRT-1), which, in mammalian cells, acts as a key regulator of energy homeostasis, gene silencing, and genomic stability, metabolism, and cell survival. The SIRT-1 is expressed in human oocytes and the nuclei of granulosa cells at several points in the developmental stages and is known to suppress inflammation. Resveratrol also protects oocytes from aging deficiency, through protection against oxidative stress (Rencber et al., 2018).

The effect of resveratrol and metformin on ovarian reserve and ultrastructure was researched by Rencber et al. (2018), in a study of the first of its kind. They concluded that there were no significant differences between the actions of resveratrol and Metformin, and that resveratrol showed superior action in reducing plasma AMH levels. This serves to indicate that resveratrol may be used alone as an alternative to Metformin, or in combination with low-dose Metformin in treatment of PCOS. Resveratrol was found to reduce inflammation in PCOS via SIRT-1 activation, alone, or in combination with Metformin. Furthermore, the researchers were optimistic that because resveratrol did not induce the side effects of Metformin (nausea, vomiting and gastro-intestinal effects), the dosage for optimal treatment could be accurately evaluated in future. However, more research in this field is needed (Rencber et al., 2018).

A randomized, double-blind, and placebo-controlled study observed that a resveratrol dosage of 600mg per day for 3 months (in patients with NAFLD), reduced their insulin resistance (HOMA-IR), glucose, total cholesterol, LDL, and liver enzymes. Resveratrol also decreased TNF-α and increased adiponectin levels, both of which are respectively important pro-inflammatory and anti-inflammatory cytokines. Although some studies did not find any benefit from resveratrol with regards to metabolic markers, this might be due to inadequate dosage. In higher dosages, resveratrol has shown the capacity to mimic the metabolic effects of caloric restriction. Furthermore, SIRT-1 seems to reduce the inflammation caused by interleukin-1β (IL-1β) in human adipose tissue, reducing the expression of other inflammatory cytokines, such as TNF-α and interleukin-8 (IL-8) Other findings demonstrated that resveratrol could reduce pro-inflammatory cytokines such as IL-6 in TNF-α-induced atherogenic changes in adipocytes, suggesting that resveratrol has beneficial effects on metabolic profiles in human obesity (Figueiredo et al., 2018).

4.5. FOLIC ACID

4.5.1. Overview of Folate and Folic Acid

Folic acid is part of the B-vitamin family, referred to as Vitamin B9, and occurs in several forms. *Folate* occurs naturally in food, circulates in the blood stream, and is found in red blood cells. *Folic acid* is the synthetic form of folate, and is used in oral supplements, and to fortify food. Folic acid is easier for the body to utilise than natural folate (Chavarro et al., 2008). The reason for this is that folate needs to undergo a methylation process in order to form methylfolate, which is the most metabolically active form of folate (Rowe, 2019; Peter-Ross et al., 2015). The gene involved in this process is known as methylenetetrahydrofolate (MTHFR). A common mutation of this gene is carried by 40% of individuals in some ethnic groups (notably more in Asian countries than in the US, Australia or New Zealand), which is associated with impaired methylation of folate and impaired folate utilization (Rowe, 2019; Gaysina, 2018).

Since the early 1990s, folic acid supplementation in pre-conceptional women was found to reduce the occurrence and re-occurrence of neural tube defects. This led to both the general recommendation of folic acid supplements to reproductive-aged females, and the folic acid fortification of food, such as bread and cereals, in many countries. The main functions of folic acid are the synthesis of DNA, transfer ribonucleic acid or RNA (our genetic material) and the production of the two amino acids, methionine and cysteine (Gaskins et al., 2012).

4.5.2. Dietary Need for Folic Acid

In 1996, the Institute of Medicine introduced a unit, known as the dietary folate equivalent (DFE):

- 1 microgram (mcg) of natural folate provides 1 mcg of DFE.
- 1 mcg of folic acid taken with meals or fortified food provides 1.7 mcg of DFE.
- 1 mcg of a folic acid supplement taken without food provides 2 mcg of DFE. (Chavarro et al., 2008, p.128).

Since reproduction is a time of extraordinary DNA replication and protein assembly, an adequate supply of folate in the bloodstream ensures that the egg and developing embryo receive sufficient amounts of this essential nutrient (Chavarro et al., 2008). In several animal studies, supplemental folic acid has resulted in increased ovulation rates, while folic acid deficiency decreased ovulation. Several previous studies have found that supplemental folic acid has an inverse relation to anovulatory infertility, and seems to have superior effects with regards to reproduction, than natural folate (Chavarro et al., 2008; Gaskins et al, 2012).

In cases of low folate, the ovarian response to FSH pulses showed impaired ovulation, and women who carry the gene mutation of MTHFR (T allele in position 677 of the MTHFR gene) have decreased ovarian responsiveness to FSH, and fewer retrievable oocytes. In animals, folate depletion has been shown to cause depleted ovarian granulosa cells, and decreased levels of progesterone. The researchers concluded that folate deficiency might lead to an "abortive" attempt at cell reproduction (Gaskins et al., 2012).

The explanation for the superior action of synthetic folic acid over natural folate, could be attributed to better absorption rates of synthetic folate. The DFE system attempts to address this issue, but it is known to be flawed. Relative to synthetic folic acid, folate from natural food has a lower proportion of absorbable and available folate. Other luminal factors may also hinder the absorption of natural folate, including destruction in the gastrointestinal tract, poor release from food matrix, and other factors that hinder absorption. Folic acid fortified foods are usually associated with additional Vitamin B12 and other micro nutrients, which could improve bioavailability of the synthetic folate (Gaskins et al., 2012).

4.5.3. Recommendations

Females in their childbearing years should consume at least 400 mcg of folic acid daily, in addition to what is provided in their diet. Pregnant women need at least 600 mcg in supplemental form, over and above their dietary intake (Chavarro et al., 2008). Most pregnancy supplements today provide at least 400 mcg folic acid per supplemental dose, with some as high as 1

000 mcg (Rowe, 2019). Table 6 below lists some foods that are rich in folic acid.

Table 6. Foods rich in folate/folic acid

Food	Serving	Dietary Folate Equivalents
Fortified breakfast cereals	¾ to 1 cup	200 – 800 mcg
White rice, enriched, cooked	1 cup	215 mcg
Lentils, cooked	½ cup	179 mcg
Pasta, cooked	1 cup	167 mcg
Garbanzo beans, cooked	½ cup	141 mcg
Spinach, cooked	½ cup	131 mcg
Asparagus, cooked	½ cup (6 spears)	121 mcg
Orange juice from concentrate (not recommended for frequent use in PCOS)	1 cup	110 mcg
Pita bread	1 piece	99 mcg
Lima beans, cooked	½ cup	78 mcg
Wheat bread	2 slices	28 mcg

Source: Chavarro et al., 2008.

4.6. VITAMIN D

Although Vitamin D seems to have therapeutic implications in improving the hormonal and metabolic biomarkers in PCOS, conflicting evidence has been found in this regard.

Vitamin D therapy normalises the elevated serum AMH in women with PCOS, and as such, could be linked to improved folliculogenesis. In contrast, a meta-analysis which reviewed the role of Vitamin D in PCOS, found no evidence of improved metabolic and hormonal indices in PCOS (Saleem & Rizvi, 2017).

Rather, a deficiency of Vitamin D may be one of the co-morbidities of PCOS. While Vitamin D deficiency might be detrimental to fertility, there is uncertainty whether higher levels of Vitamin D might provide additional benefit, once sufficiency has been reached (Gaskins & Chavarro, 2018).

4.7. ADIPONECTIN

Low levels of adiponectin, seem to connect PCOS, obesity and insulin resistance, with an inverse relationship between adiponectin and IR. The hormones produced by adipose tissue (adipokines), such as adiponectin, play an important role in limiting androgen production from the ovaries. The drugs that are being developed to target the stimulation of adiponectin for management of metabolic and cardio-vascular dysfunction, may also provide a therapeutic benefit for females suffering from PCOS (Saleem & Rizvi, 2017).

Measuring adiponectin levels can also be helpful as a biomarker in young, lean women with PCOS or in women with a family history of PCOS. The mechanism of adiponectin action is probably a reduction in the expression of adiponectin receptors in the theca cells of PCOS females, due to the defective action of adiponectin. In animals, theca cells treated with adiponectin, presented a significant reduction in gene expression of the key androgen synthesis enzymes. It is still uncertain whether the changes in adiponectin receptors are a cause or a consequence of obesity or IR (Saleem & Rizvi, 2017).

Quercetin, one of the many flavonoids (a diverse group of plant chemicals responsible for the bright colours, are powerful anti-oxidants with anti-inflammatory properties and benefits to the immune system) found in plants, and one of the most abundant overall, (Figueiredo et al., 2018), was found to increase the levels of adiponectin by 5.56%, and found to favour adiponectin-mediated insulin sensitivity in PCOS. While rodent models have demonstrated promise in improvement in PCOS phenotype, evidence for its benefit is still lacking. Adiponectin is utilized better as a biomarker than a treatment option in patients with PCOS (Saleem & Rizvi, 2017).

4.8. Fatty Acids

4.8.1. Overview of Fatty Acids

As already discussed, chronic insulin resistance appears to be directly or indirectly related to diet-induced inflammation, of which the mechanisms at molecular level are manifold and complex. These mechanisms are based on the ability of cellular inflammation to interrupt the action of insulin by disrupting signaling mechanisms. Interestingly, the notion that inflammation may be related to IR came more than a century ago when the observation was made that anti-inflammatory drugs, such as salicylates and aspirin, were effective in reducing hyperglycemia in diabetes (Sears & Perry, 2015).

Much of the IR that characterizes metabolic dysfunction, may be diet-induced, via the role of various fatty acids. Both omega-3 (Ω-3) and omega-6 (Ω-6) fatty acids are long-chain poly-unsaturated fatty acids (PUFA) and are essential fats to the human body. They are not inter-convertible, and are metabolically distinct, with opposing physiological effects, making balance between these two fatty acids in the human diet of great importance (Figueiredo et al., 2018).

Arachidonic acid (AA), a polyunsaturated fat, is the active end-product of enzyme action on the primary Ω-6 fatty acid, linoleic acid, and is viewed as a strong inflammatory molecule (together with palmitic acid, which is a saturated fatty acid). Eicosapentanoic acid (EPA) and docosahexanoic acid (DHA) are the active end products of enzyme action on the primary Ω-3 fat, α-linolenic acid. EPA and DHA can be viewed as anti-inflammatory polyunsaturated fats because they have the ability to generate substances and binding proteins that are able to decrease IR within an organ (Sears & Perry, 2015).

In various ways, IR seems to start in the hypothalamus. Excessive inflammatory fat, such as AA, palmitic acid, or an excess of caloric intake, can inflame the hypothalamus, leading to resistance to the satiety signaling of both insulin and leptin, which results in reduced satiety and increased hunger. The hypothalamus also contains binding proteins that respond specifically to long-chain omega-3 fatty acids such as EPA and DHA, decreasing the inflammation in the hypothalamus (Sears & Perry, 2015).

The current western diet is known to contain excessive amounts of Ω-6 PUFAs with low levels of Ω-3 PUFAs, leading to an unhealthy ratio of Ω-6 to Ω-3 of around 20 : 1, instead of 1 : 1, which is the ratio that had been consumed throughout evolution (Figueiredo et al., 2018). Omega-3 PUFAs also metabolically compete with Ω-6 PUFAs, so that a diet high in α-6 fatty acids promotes deficient Ω-3 PUFA intake even further (Grassi, 2013).

4.8.2. Supplementation of Fatty Acids

Supplementation with α-3 fats may be helpful for improving IR, BMI and hirsutism in females with PCOS. A dosage of 1 500 mg per day of α-3 for at least six months, showed improvements in LH, testosterone, and SHBG levels. Since α-3 supplementation has been shown to be helpful in the treatment of infertility, patients should be advised by registered dieticians and other well-informed professionals about foods rich in α-3 fatty acids, specifically EPA and DHA, such as fatty fish and supplementation with these fats. Fish oil supplements are generally tolerated well, and the US Food and Drug Administration (FDA) has concluded that up to 4g per day is generally regarded as safe (GRAS). Larger dosages may cause bleeding by inhibiting platelet aggregation (Grassi, 2013).

In consultation with a well-informed registered dietician, the issue of fatty acid supplementation should be discussed with the PCOS patient. Guidance should be given as to eating at least 100g of fatty fish twice a week, but also discussing other options of increasing α-3 intake. Not all supplements provide good quantities of EPA/DHA in one or two capsules, so choosing the correct supplement without wasting financial resources, is an important conversation to have with the PCOS patient.

Chapter 5

PCOS IN ADOLESCENCE

5.1. OVERVIEW

It is critical that energy stores in the young developing female are sufficient to support the attainment of reproductive maturation, and maintenance of fertility in adulthood. Conditions of severe energy depletion, such as excessive exercise, anorexia nervosa, as well as the contrary, such as extreme energy surplus in obesity, can lead to delayed or absent pubertal onset in adolescents and infertility in adulthood (Nomair et al., 2014).

Early lifestyle intervention, especially in pre-pubertal girls at risk for PCOS and young adolescents with PCOS, has been shown to improve metabolic, reproductive, and endocrine parameters. This appears to be mediated through normalization of the neuro-peptides in the arcuate nucleus of the hypothalamus, as well as regulation of the neuro-peptides in the HPO-axis (Saleem & Rizvi, 2017).

Although PCOS often presents in the vulnerable stage of puberty/adolescence, there are several barriers to accurate diagnosis and treatment, as some features of PCOS and MS overlap during the normal progression of puberty. There are also no universally-accepted criteria for diagnosis of PCOS in adolescence, although a few suggestions have been put forward, which are helpful in clinical practice (Agapova et al., 2014;

Orsino, Van Eyk & Hamilton, 2005; Reinehr et al., 2017; Roe & Dokras, 2011).

Recognition of PCOS in adolescents allows for early screening for any existing metabolic complications, and early intervention and treatment, which would reduce the morbidity of the condition, as well as the psychological and financial burdens later in life. Adolescents with PCOS also show significantly lower scores on self-esteem and quality of life. Therefore, further research is needed to determine the role of treatment of the condition to improve the psychological stress among young PCOS women (Grassi, 2013; Orsino et al., 2005).

5.2. Investigations and Diagnosis of PCOS in Adolescence

Adolescent PCOS women usually have several complaints when seeking medical help, including irregular menses, hirsutism, acne, and weight concerns. Depending on the specialist from which the medical attention is sought, there are differences in approaches between endocrinologists and gynaecologists and general practitioners. There are currently no evidence-based guidelines with regards to appropriate investigations in adolescent women suspected of having PCOS, and it is suggested that investigation starts with tests to exclude other endocrinopathies which might mimic PCOS (Orsino et al., 2005).

Different diagnostic criteria have been put forward by different authors. In 2006, researchers Sultan and Paris (as cited by Roe & Dokras, 2011) recommended that adolescent girls meet four out of five of the following criteria before being diagnosed with PCOS:

- Oligo- or amenorrhea longer than two years after menarche (onset of menses);
- Clinical hyperandrogenism;
- Biological hyperandrogenism;

- Hyperinsulinemia or insulin resistance;
- Polycystic morphology of the ovaries on ultrasonic examination.

Another suggestion by different researchers is to apply the Rotterdam criteria (androgen excess, irregular menses, ovarian polycystic morphology), but that diagnosis is only definitive if all three criteria are met. These researchers also suggested that, for those exhibiting two out of the three criteria, PCOS may well be diagnosed in adulthood, and these subjects should be followed up and re-evaluated on a regular basis (Agapova et al., 2014; Roe & Dokras, 2011).

5.2.1. Androgen Excess

Most studies agree that 65% of adolescents with PCOS present with hirsutism. Acne, in contrast, occurs at a high rate (69%) in healthy adolescence, which precludes its use as a marker of hyperandrogenism in PCOS. Alopecia due to androgen excess has not been studied sufficiently in this population and seems unimportant for the purpose of assessment for PCOS. Consequently, the most useful marker of clinical hyperandrogenism in screening for PCOS in adolescence is hirsutism (Agapova et al., 2014; Roe & Dokras, 2011).

5.2.2. Irregular Menses

Because the HPO-axis undergoes progressive development over a period of several years after menarche, the menstrual pattern might be difficult to distinguish from anovulation during puberty. It was also found that 55% of menstrual cycles, during the first two years after menarche, are anovulatory. Although irregular menses cannot be used as the only criterion for PCOS in adolescence, its persistence after two years post menarche, is cause for concern regarding PCOS (Agapova et al., 2014; Roe & Dokras, 2011).

Evidence exists that a greater irregularity of the menstrual cycle is associated with a more severe phenotype of PCOS, and higher levels of excess androgens. Adolescents with amenorrhea have more features of MS and higher levels of androgens, than those with oligomenorrhea. Body mass index (BMI) and menstrual history, are reliable predictors of continuing amenorrhea (Agapova et al., 2014). A suggested definition of adolescent ovulatory dysfunction is the absence of menstruation for longer than 90 days, or continuing cycles longer than 45 days. Menstrual irregularity should be further investigated in adolescents when it presents for longer than one year, and is associated with other signs of symptoms of PCOS (Agapova et al., 2014).

5.2.3. Ovarian Polycystic Morphology

Many healthy adolescents show polycystic ovaries on ultrasonic examination, making this marker of little value as a diagnostic criterion for PCOS (Agapova et al., 2014; Roe & Dokras, 2011). Ovarian volume and appearance vary during adolescence, and polycystic or enlarged ovaries may well become normal over time. Most importantly, the ultrasonic examination of the ovaries in adolescents should be done trans-abdominally, especially in virginal adolescents, where transvaginal examination would be inappropriate. However, trans-abdominal ultrasonic examinations are less accurate, especially in obese patients, who comprise half of the PCOS population (Agapova et al., 2014; Roe & Dokras, 2011).

5.3. OBESITY, INSULIN RESISTANCE AND METABOLIC RISK

After diagnosis of the adolescent with PCOS, she should be screened for associated metabolic dysfunctions. Acanthosis nigricans and abdominal obesity are clinical pointers towards insulin resistance. One third (33%) of adolescents with PCOS meet some of the criteria for MS, as opposed to five percent (5%) of adolescents without PCOS. The Pediatric Adult Treatment Panel III diagnostic criteria for metabolic syndrome in adolescents require three out of five (3/5) of the following to apply (Roe & Dokras, 2011):

- Blood glucose > 100 mg/dl (5.5 mmol/l);
- HDL-C (high-density lipoprotein cholesterol) < 40 mg/dl (2.2 mmol/l);
- Triglycerides > 110 mg/dl (6.1 mmol/l);
- Waist circumference >/= 90th percentile for age and sex;
- Blood pressure >/= 90th percentile for age and sex.

Although obesity is prevalent amongst adolescent PCOS, it does not fully explain the other metabolic characteristics associated with PCOS. Impaired glucose tolerance (IGT) is found at an increased rate in adolescents diagnosed with PCOS, and is associated with insulin resistance and a strong predictor of T2DM, CVD and early death. The incidence of IGT amongst the adolescent PCOS population is as high as 30%, but impaired fasting glucose and T2DM can also present. Screening by using an oral glucose tolerance test (OGTT) is more sensitive than just using fasting glucose, and at the same time, screens for T2DM (Agapova et al., 2014; Orsino et al., 2005). Although the studies on adolescent PCOS are still relatively small, the need for regular screening using an OGTT and complete lipid profile is strongly recommended by the AE-PCOS Society (Roe & Dokras, 2011).

5.4. TREATMENT OF PCOS IN ADOLESCENCE

As with treatment of adult PCOS, the first line of therapy should always include weight loss and lifestyle management. Secondary treatments such as Metformin and oral contraceptives could be considered as secondary treatments for improvement of symptoms. Further research into the diagnostic criteria for PCOS in the adult population is needed before consensus can be reached about appropriate pharmacological treatment, so as not to result in premature use of drugs in a condition that might not be fully diagnosed. In addition, the many points of overlap between normal developmental puberty and the features of PCOS, suggest that a more conservative approach to diagnosis of PCOS in adolescents should be considered, compared to diagnosis of PCOS in adults (Agapova et al., 2014).

In 2017, Thomas Reinehr and his team performed a longitudinal study of obese girls with and without PCOS, in a one-year lifestyle intervention to evaluate the relationship between AMH, weight status, and androgens. They concluded that AMH levels in adolescent girls with PCOS were conclusively higher than in girls without PCOS. Higher AMH levels were consistent with higher LH and androgen levels. The high AMH levels in the PCOS group normalised together with weight loss, which probably suggested a decrease in antral follicle number. The researchers also reported that a longer period of intervention is required for adequate reductions in AMH to manifest (Reinehr et al., 2017).

The researchers used "The Obeldicks concept", as the method of lifestyle intervention (Dobe et al., 2011) for this study (Reinehr et al., 2017). This lifestyle intervention is of German origin and comprises a one-year intervention for obese children aged eight to sixteen (8 to 16 years). "Obeldicks Light" is a six-month intervention for the same age group of overweight children, and "Obeldicks Mini" is a one-year intervention for obese children aged four to seven (4 to 7 years). Obeldicks is based on nutritional education, physical activity, behaviour therapy and individual psychological therapy and care.

The Obeldicks intervention has proven successful in the following areas:

- Low dropout rate;
- Reduced BMI;
- Improved glucose tolerance and metabolism;
- Significant improvement of hypertension and dyslipidemia.

The quality of life of the participants was significantly improved, and the achieved weight loss was sustained four years after the end of the intervention. Training manuals and seminars for professionals aid in the implementation of the Obeldicks lifestyle interventions (Dobe et al., 2011).

Part II:
Nutritional Considerations and Treatment Strategies for the Woman with PCOS

Chapter 6

THE OPTIMAL DIET FOR PCOS

6.1. A HISTORICAL OVERVIEW

The basic goal for the treatment of PCOS was, and still is, to restore fertility through normalising of serum androgen levels, which can only be achieved when insulin resistance is reduced by decreasing the total body weight, and the abdominal/visceral fat of the patient (Moran & Norman, 2004). Improvement in insulin sensitivity and reduction of hyperinsulinemia are recognised as the core reasons for bringing about improvement in metabolic and reproductive outcomes, which suggest that dietary manipulation that is designed to improve IR might be of greater benefit than merely restricting energy intake (Douglas et al., 2006, Farshchi et al., 2007, Marsh & Brand-Miller, 2005). Although several studies have alluded to weight loss as the cornerstone of dietary treatment for the obese PCOS patient, a myriad of different approaches have been suggested over more than a decade, to achieve the desired weight loss. Among the approaches have been the following:

- Energy restriction (Herriott et al., 2008; Marsh & Brand-Miller, 2005; Sikaris, 2004);
- Modifications in macronutrient contents (differing ratios between fat, carbohydrate and protein) (Douglas et al., 2006, Sikaris, 2004);

- Reduction of the glycemic index (GI) and the glycemic load (GL) of carbohydrate intake (Herriott et al., 2008; Marsh & Brand-Miller, 2005; Moran & Norman, 2004);
- Decrease in the saturated and trans-fat contents, and modification of the monounsaturated fat content of the diet (Douglas et al., 2006, Chavarro et al., 2007b, Farshchi et al., 2007); and
- Meal replacement used as a short-term strategy (Moran et al., 2006).

Weight loss prior to pregnancy also improves live birth rate in obese women, regardless of PCOS. Weight loss is internationally recommended and accepted as the first-line therapy in obese women with PCOS who wish to become pregnant (Thessaloniki workshop group, 2008). The benefits of weight loss have been demonstrated in such conditions as diabetes and CVD, and obesity is well recognised for its association with poor fertility outcome. Several studies have shown that improved spontaneous ovulation is associated with as little as 5% weight loss in females who suffer from PCOS. Weight loss of 5% to 10% of initial body weight has been shown in studies to be associated with improved insulin sensitivity and reduction in circulating insulin levels, as well as reduction in hyperandrogenism with improvement of menstrual function, ovulation and fertility, and hirsutism (Farshchi et al., 2007; Moran et al., 2004). Although the reproductive function resumes with weight loss of as little as 10% of initial body weight, the BMI of the PCOS sufferer having lost weight might still be above $30 kg/m^2$ (Moran et al., 2004). Siebert, Kruger and Lombard (2009) showed that the "ideal" BMI for successful reproductive outcome in PCOS, whether drug-intervention was necessary or not, is $27 kg/m^2$.

After more than two decades of research, the exact nature of the dietary manipulations to bring about favourable reproductive outcome, or improvement in symptoms of PCOS is still unclear (Douglas et al., 2006; Marsh & Brand-Miller, 2005; Moran & Norman, 2004; Thessaloniki workshop group, 2008). This is attributed to limited literature and lack of long-term randomized controlled trials (RCTs), and confusing, conflicting findings (Grassi, 2013).

The 'standard diet' that most of research based its findings on was the universally-known and accepted high fiber diet, which has low fat (no more than 30% of total calories), moderate protein (15% of total calories) and high carbohydrates (50% of total calories) (Moran et al., 2013). Since this distribution of nutrients had been ingrained in all students of nutrition and hailed as the 'standard diet' with which, by suggestion, no harm could be done, slight variations in macro-nutrient ratios and applying the standard diet as such, but with caloric deficit, really remained the only options.

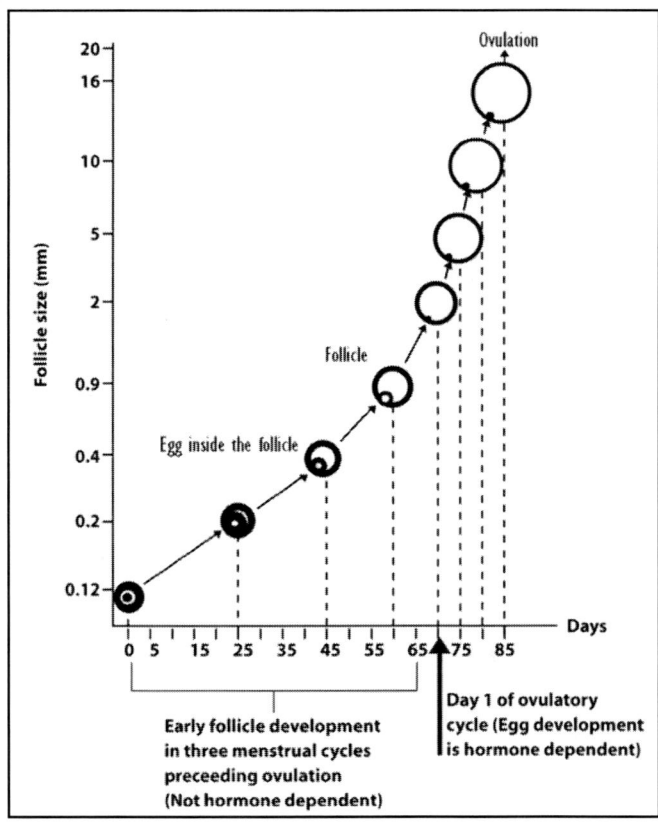

Source: Gougeon, 1996, cited by Silber, 2018.

Figure 11. Ovarian follicle: 85 days of development.

In 2007, the Thessaloniki workshop group, held in Greece suggested a combination of therapies, including behavioural counselling, diet and exercise, pharmacological treatment and bariatric surgery. They also cautioned that energy restriction, increased physical activity, and agents to induce weight loss may be harmful to the fetus in the peri-conception period. Hence it was advised that such interventions should probably not take place together with fertility treatment, but prior thereto, until the risk of the therapies for pregnancy are better understood. This correlates well with the fact that primordial cells, after "awakening", take up to 70 days to respond to menstrual hormones, to develop and reach their full potential at roughly 85 days. Therefore, the dietary treatment and lifestyle improvements for the female with PCOS seeking fertility should start at least 3 to 4 months before administering any drugs or other medical intervention used in fertility enhancement, by which time it is hoped and probable that the female would have fallen pregnant spontaneously. Figure 11 shows the development of the ovarian follicle over 85 days.

The Thessaloniki workshop group of 2008 referred to the "Atkins Diet" and very-low-calorie-diets, which seemed to have been able to decrease body weight by 12% in 24 weeks, and improved reproductive outcome. They also mentioned that diets with reduced glycemic load (amount of carbohydrate) seemed to be beneficial to alleviate insulin resistance and its metabolic consequences, and concluded by saying: "…the recommended diet for obese women with PCOS is any hypocaloric diet (with a 500kcal per day deficit) with reduced glycemic load, and, failing that, any calorie-restricted diet with which patients can comply and achieve a 5% weight loss".

In 2009, Moran et al. published a literature review on the treatment of obesity in PCOS, as a position statement of the Androgen Excess and Polycystic Ovary Syndrome (AE-PCOS) Society. They agreed on the following:

- Lifestyle modification should be the first line of therapy in treating PCOS.
- Energy reduction by 500 to 1000kcal per day could be effective options for weight loss, assisting in a loss of 7% to 12% of initial body weight over 6 to 12 months.

- Dietary regimes should be nutritionally complete, and appropriate for life stage, citing fat contents of less than 30% of total energy intake, and saturated fat of less than 10% total energy intake, with adequate fiber from whole grain cereals, fruit and vegetables.
- Alternative dietary options (reducing carbohydrate and increasing protein) may be successful, but more research is needed.
- Structure and support within a weight-management regime is crucial and might even outweigh the importance of dietary composition.
- Aim for at least 30 minutes of structured, moderate exercise per day.

Moran et al. (2009) concluded with the undeniable benefits of weight loss to improve reproductive health and metabolic status, but also the question as to how to increase program retention (reduce dropout) and secure long-term maintenance of lost weight. "There are no studies on long-term weight regain after lifestyle intervention with or without anti-obesity drugs or surgery in overweight or obese PCOS patients. This remains an open question that should be investigated" (Moran et al., 2009).

In 2013, Moran and colleagues published a systematic review on the optimal diet composition for the treatment of PCOS. Five different dietary interventions were followed, after which the researchers concluded that the presentation of PCOS is improved with weight loss, regardless of the dietary composition.

Katoaka and colleagues (2017) performed a systematic review of weight management interventions in women with PCOS, and were the first to do this in comparison to matched subjects without PCOS. They noted that women with PCOS seem to gain weight faster, and have a higher prevalence of overweight, compared to the non-PCOS counterparts. They also suggested that weight management interventions in women with PCOS may be less effective compared to those without PCOS, because of the higher rate of longitudinal weight gain in women with PCOS. This might also be related to hormonal dysregulation in PCOS or the presence of IR, contributing to abnormalities in energy homeostasis and appetite regulation, or to the reduced post-prandial thermogenesis seen in females with PCOS.

Katoaka and colleagues (2017) identified 14 studies, including 933 women with considerable clinical heterogeneity, across a range of lifestyle and non-lifestyle interventions for weight management, and found no significant differences in the weight changes between PCOS and non-PCOS women at the end of each intervention. In previous studies, it has been shown that women with PCOS have a higher caloric intake and tendency towards eating junk food, which corresponds to the higher rate of weight gain. The researchers reported that the studies were small, and the dropout rate was high. Much more research into appetite control and self-regulation around food among PCOS women and non-PCOS women is needed.

For lean or normal-weight PCOS women, very little is available in literature about dietary changes, but this group of PCOS women still presents with abdominal fat accumulation (Herriott et al., 2009), and the underlying insulin resistance and inflammation which are typical of PCOS as already described. The dietary entities of concern, that are described in Section 6.4 (trans fats, lowering the glycemic load of their diet, consuming full-fat milk, AGEs, and fructose excess, etc.) are as relevant for the lean PCOS population as it is for the overweight PCOS population. One might suggest that lean PCOS women implement the single guidelines as such into an improved, consistent balanced diet, while maintaining caloric intake adequate to sustain normal weight.

6.2. THE NURSES' HEALTH STUDY

6.2.1. Nurses' Health Study: Original Cohort

The Nurses' Health Study (NHS) was established by Dr. Frank Speizer in 1976 with continuous funding from the National Institutes of Health since that time. The primary motivation for the study was to investigate the potential long-term consequences of oral contraceptives, which were being prescribed to hundreds of millions of women.

The Nurses' Health Study (NHS) and the Nurses' Health Study II (NHS II) are among the largest prospective investigations into the risk factors for major chronic diseases in women. Former Secretary of the US Department of Health and Human Services, Donna Shalala, called the NHS "one of the most significant studies ever conducted on the health of women" (NHS, 2018).

6.2.2. Why Nurses?

Nurses were selected as the study population because of their knowledge about health and their ability to provide complete and accurate information regarding various diseases, due to their nursing education.

NHS founders anticipated and found that nurses were able to respond with a high degree of accuracy to brief, technically-worded questionnaires. They were relatively easy to follow over time and were motivated to participate in a long-term study. The cohort was limited to married women due to the sensitivity of questions about contraceptive use at that time.

6.2.3. Establishing the Cohort

Married registered nurses, aged 30 to 55 in 1976, who lived in the 11 most populous states, and whose nursing boards agreed to supply NHS with their members' names and addresses, were eligible to be enrolled in the cohort if they responded to the NHS baseline questionnaire. The original states were California, Connecticut, Florida, Maryland, Massachusetts, Michigan, New Jersey, New York, Ohio, Pennsylvania, and Texas (NHS, 2018).

Originally, the focus of the Nurses' Health Study was on contraception, smoking, cancer and heart disease, but over time the study grew to include research over many other lifestyle factors and behaviours, and in excess of 30 diseases.

The Nurses' Health Study II (NHS II) was established by Dr. Walter Willett and colleagues in 1989 with NIH funding, with the focus of studying contraception, diet, and lifestyle risk factors, identifying a study population younger than the original NHS cohort.

In 2010, the NHS III was established by Dr. Jorge Chavarro, Dr. Walter Willett, Dr. Janet Rich-Edwards, and Dr. Stacey Missmer. The researchers found importance in including nurses from more diverse ethnic backgrounds, and the NHS III was focused on how dietary patterns, lifestyle, environment, and nursing occupational exposures impact on their health. Women's health issues around new hormone treatments and fertility/pregnancy, as well as adolescent diet and breast cancer risk were examined (NHS, 2018).

The NHS has contributed valuable information towards women's health, also in the field of fertility/infertility and nutrition.

6.3. Dropout

Lifestyle intervention in a free-living society, can never be exact or flawless, due to the many choices and temptations that surround women who live in families, being the caretaker or cook for their family, and having to procure food through supermarkets with endless choices and manipulations to falter. The sustainability of weight reduction diets in obese women with PCOS is well known to be poor over the long term, with little maintenance of weight loss (Huber-Buchholz et al., 1999). Moran et al. (2006) substantiated the view by referring to the 26% to 38% dropout rate for PCOS sufferers on weight-loss regimes, as opposed to the 8% to 9% in non-PCOS subjects.

Weidemann (2012) studied 86 females seeking help at the Infertility Clinic of the Tygerberg Hospital in Cape Town, South Africa. They were diagnosed with PCOS according to the Rotterdam criteria, and had a BMI of more than 27kg/m^2. The women signed consent to attend three visits with the dietician, the initial assessment and education, and two follow-up visits, spanning a period of 3 months. After the first visit, 50% of the subjects had dropped out of the study, and after the second visit 41% of the remaining subjects, had also dropped out. Only 18 out of 86 initial recruitments could be studied, at the end of the study, due to the high dropout rate. Interestingly, a questionnaire at baseline showed that none of the women in the study had ever tried diet or improved lifestyle as a way to lose weight, but rather resorted to 'diet herbs and teas', appetite suppressants and other alternative medicines to assist in weight loss. All the subjects reported failure at their own attempts at weight loss (Weidemann, 2012).

Recently, a large RCT in the Netherlands, randomized 600 infertile obese females to a 6-month lifestyle intervention, prior to 18 months of fertility treatment, or immediate fertility treatment for 24 months. The dropout rate in the lifestyle intervention group was 21.8%, which, as has been mentioned, is an issue in weight loss studies. The primary outcome of the study was term vaginal birth rate within 24 months, which was significantly higher in the immediate treatment group, which raised the question of whether fertility treatment should be delayed. The spontaneous pregnancy rate, however, was higher in the intervention group. The researchers also reminded the reader that weight loss before conception in the obese population, ameliorates risks in pregnancy. Many studies have also shown the negative impact of obesity on ART outcomes, where the smaller oocytes are less likely to fertilize normally, and also that live birth rates correlate negatively with increasing BMI (Broughton & Moley, 2017).

Although anecdotal reports of increased difficulty with weight loss in PCOS abound, the phenomenon has never been scientifically proven. Some studies have suggested increased difficulty with weight loss in PCOS, and as mentioned, that this might be the result of longitudinal weight gain. The high dropout rate among PCOS sufferers might also be due to abnormal appetite regulation, leading to difficulty with energy restriction. This implies that PCOS is a population that requires intensive long-term dietary coaching, with regular follow-up and support. Dietary strategies to maximise satiety are certainly applicable to help the patients to achieve a desirable body weight (Moran et al., 2006).

6.4. Dietary Entities of Concern to PCOS Nutrition

6.4.1. Trans Fat

As already mentioned, Chavarro et al. (2007b) conducted a trial lasting 8 years, including 18 500 subjects from the NHS, and examined the association between the intakes of different types of fat and ovulatory infertility. The researchers found that the consumption of trans-fatty acids, instead of carbohydrates, monounsaturates or omega-6 polyunsaturates, was associated with greater risk of ovulatory infertility. Intake of trans-fatty acids is also associated with increased concentrations of inflammatory markers, and with greater insulin resistance and risk for type-2 diabetes mellitus (T2DM). Women planning to become pregnant should receive advice regarding their fat intake to improve their overall risk for CVD and diabetes, although responding well to such advice could also serve to improve their fertility (Chavarro et al., 2007b).

Trans fats have been of concern to public health for over 3 decades. Originally launched by Procter and Gamble in 1911, the "frenzy" over margarine started with claims such as "it's vegetable, it's digestible!", including cookbooks and appealing to the kosher community who had been waiting for thousands of years for a non-dairy fat (Khazan, 2013). Decades would pass, until the inflammatory nature of trans fats would be recognized, and the FDA proposed changing its classification of trans fats to no longer be "generally regarded as safe" (GRAS), on June 15, 2015. The notion that trans fats had been "banned" by the FDA is incorrect – it was merely removed from the GRAS list. The FDA gave food manufacturers 3 years to remove trans fats from their products or submit a petition for the inclusion of trans fats in their product, with a 3-year deadline. From the early 1980s into the 1990s, the health risks of trans fats began to surface, especially their participation in increased CVD risk. Today, it is estimated that trans fats may have contributed to thousands of early deaths, and the threshold for "safe" intake of trans fat, even as low as less than 1% of daily total energy, is undetermined and still in the process of debate (Peterson & Zu, 2016). Table 7 gives some insight into the trans-fat contents of different foods.

In their study of dietary fatty acids and the risk of ovulatory infertility, Chavarro et al. (2007b) found that the intake of polyunsaturated fatty acids was not protective in their entire study group of the NHS at the time.

Table 7. Trans-fat contents of food

Trans-fat contents in various foods, ranked in grams per 100g	
Food type	Trans-fat content
shortenings	10 to 33g
margarine, spreads	0.2 to 26g
butter	2 to 7g
cookies and crackers	1 to 8g
breads/cake products	0.1 to 10g
cake frostings, sweets	0.1 to 7g
animal fat	0 to 5g
salty snacks	0 to 4g
ground beef	1g
whole milk	0.07 to 0.1g

Source: Tarrago-Trani et al., 2006.

Practical advice for the PCOS woman improving her dietary intake, is to read the list of ingredients on all labels carefully, looking out for the words "hydrogenated" or "partially hydrogenated" vegetable fats and also the words trans fats. These products should be avoided at all cost.

6.4.2. Glycemic Index and Glycemic Load

Improvement in insulin sensitivity and reduction of hyperinsulinemia are recognised as the core reasons for bringing about improvement in metabolic and reproductive outcomes. Therefore, dietary manipulation that is designed to improve insulin resistance might be of greater benefit than merely restricting energy intake (Douglas et al., 2006; Farshchi et al., 2007; Marsh & Brand-Miller 2005).

Increasing evidence suggests that diets with a reduced glycemic load (GL) might be beneficial in reducing hyperinsulinemia and its associated consequences (Farshchi et al., 2007; Herriot et al., 2008; Marsh & Brand-Miller, 2005; Thessaloniki workshop group, 2008). The glycemic load of carbohydrates is defined as the amount of carbohydrate in a particular food, multiplied by the GI of that food (Farshchi et al., 2007).

Glycemic index (GI) can be seen as a type of carbohydrate, while glycemic load (GL) can be seen as the amount of dietary carbohydrate consumed. Altered dietary composition may influence insulin sensitivity, even without weight loss. A reduction of the GL may reduce postprandial glycaemia and the resultant hyperinsulinemia. The best way to bring about a reduced GL remains unclear, although it *could* be either of the following two ways: reducing the GI of carbohydrate intake; or cutting down on the total amount of carbohydrate consumed (Marsh & Brand-Miller, 2005).

Jenkins et al. (1981) developed and introduced the concept of GI to facilitate the classification of carbohydrates according to their postprandial glycemic effect, although the classification was based on a very small sample of 34 subjects. The main purpose with the concept of GI was to improve glycemic control in diabetics, and a meta-analysis by Brand-Miller et al. (2005) confirmed the benefits to be obtained thereby. Moran et al., (2006) reported that the modification of the type of dietary carbohydrate or GI had been highly controversial until then, and that high carbohydrate diets (50% of total energy intake) might have worsened the metabolic profile *if no weight loss was achieved*. Although data existed that lowering the GI of dietary carbohydrate improved satiety, the evidence for weight loss was poor. In addition, there appeared to be no evidence of the usefulness of GI as a strategy for weight management in women with PCOS at the time.

After the inception of the concept of GI in 1981, it was applied to numerous health states, such as diabetes, heart disease, gastro-intestinal diseases and obesity. However, the discussion on GI in this book would be incomplete without mentioning the work of Holt, Brand-Miller and Petocz in 1997, on determining the insulin index of foods. The aim of their study was to compare the postprandial insulin responses of 240 calorie-portions (1 000kJ) of 38 common foods. They obtained finger-prick blood samples every 15 minutes over a period of 120 minutes after ingestion of the food, and calculated an insulin score from the area under the insulin response curve, much the same way in which the glycemic index was established. White bread was used as the reference, with a score of 100%.

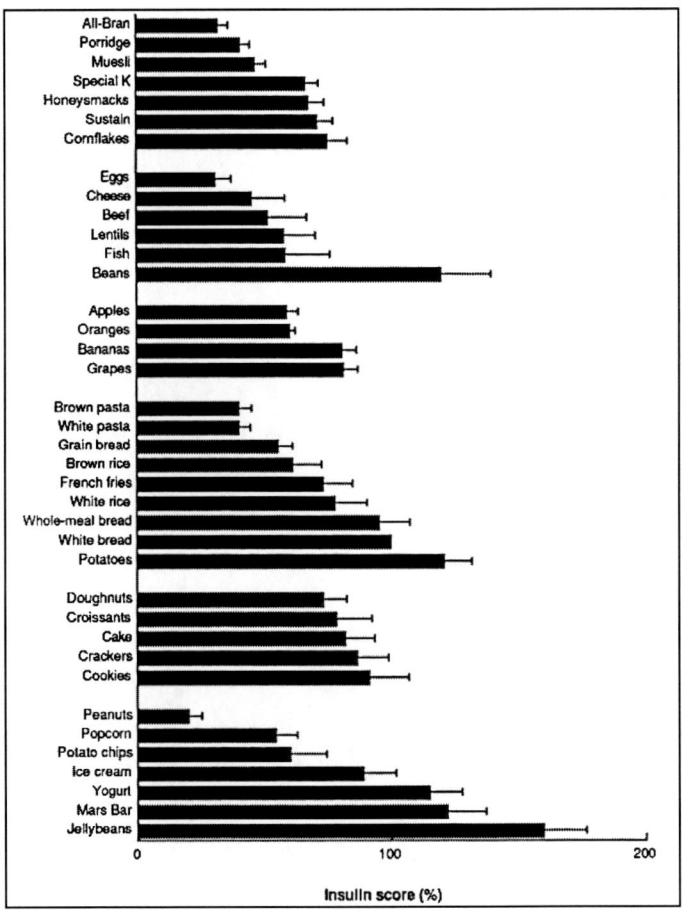

Source: Holt et al., 1997.

Figure 12. The mean insulin scores for 1000kJ (240 calorie) portions of 38 different foods.

The results of the study by Holt et al. (1997) both confirmed and challenged the basic assumptions about the relation between food intake and insulin response. Although predictably, bread and potatoes were among the most insulinogenic foods, some protein and fat-rich foods such as eggs, beef, and cheese, elicited as high an insulin response as some carbohydrate-rich foods. (Refer to Figure 12.) The fiber content of foods did not predict the magnitude of the insulin response, as white and brown pasta, and white and brown bread had much the same insulin score. Dried beans (consumed as baked beans), together with potatoes and jelly beans had the highest insulin scores. The study supported the hypothesis that the postprandial insulin response was not necessarily proportional to the glycemic response (the rise in blood sugar after consumption of food) and that other nutrients than carbohydrate affect the level of postprandial insulinemia (Holt et al., 1997).

6.4.3. Protein

Of the 20 amino acids provided by the diet for synthesis and repair, 7 are known as "essential" or "indispensible" amino acids, as they can only be obtained from food, and not manufactured from the backbones of other nutrients, like the remaining 13. In nutritional terms, protein quality refers to the ability of a single protein food to fulfil our need for essential amino acids. Animal-based proteins, such as meat, fish, poultry, eggs and dairy products, are regarded as high-quality proteins, with most products providing all 7 of the essential amino acids in one food. Plant-based proteins, such as dried beans, lentils, soya, rice, and nuts, only partially provide essential amino acids, and should be complemented with other plant proteins to obtain sufficient amounts of essential amino acids (Weidemann & Brand, 2016).

Chavarro et al. (2008) reported on the impact of protein on ovulatory infertility, from data from the NHS. They reported that women from the highest protein-intake group (115g/day) were 41% more likely to experience ovulatory infertility, compared to women from the lowest protein-intake group (77g/day), after correcting for smoking, fat intake, weight, and other factors that might influence fertility. Interestingly, ovulatory infertility was 39% more likely in women with the highest intake of animal protein, compared to those with the lowest intake. The following was found when caloric intake was kept the same:

- The addition of one serving of red meat, chicken or turkey per day, predicted an almost 30% increase in the risk of ovulatory infertility;
- The addition of one serving of fish or egg per day had no influence on ovulatory infertility;
- The addition of one serving per day of dried beans, peas, tofu or soya beans, or nuts, seemed modestly protective against ovulatory infertility.

The researchers continued to clarify these statements as follows:

- The addition of animal protein instead of carbohydrate to the diet, was related to a higher risk of an ovulatory infertility;
- The addition of plant proteins instead of carbohydrate to the diet was related to a lower risk of an ovulatory infertility;
- The addition of plant protein instead of animal protein, proved even more effective in lowering the risk of infertility.

The researchers then speculated that plant protein might be 'packaged' differently to animal protein, specifically the saturated fat content in animal protein, but also the nutrients included in the 'package'.

6.4.3.1. Iron in Protein-Rich Foods

Again, the probable explanation came from data from the NHS, which showed that the women with least difficulty with an ovulatory infertility took iron in tablet form, but that a small amount of iron did not make a difference. Larger amounts such as 80mg of iron seemed to provide the benefit. Women who received their iron from meat products, were not protected from an ovulatory infertility at all, while those taking their iron from supplements, vegetables and beans, improved their chances of getting pregnant.

Dietary iron presents itself in two forms: heme iron (such as that obtained from animal sources since heme iron is contained in red blood cells), and non-heme iron, which is mostly found in plant products such as vegetables, grains and some fruits, but also eggs and milk.

Table 8. Good sources of non-heme iron compared to some best sources of heme iron

Food	Serving size	Iron (mg)	Dietary reference intake RDA for pregnant women*
Dry fortified cereals	1 cup	-16	-59%
Soybeans, cooked	1 cup	8.8	33%
White beans, cooked	1 cup	7.8	29%
Lentils, cooked	1 cup	6.6	24%
Spinach, cooked	1 cup	6.6	24%
Beef liver, braised	3 oz	5.4	20%
Black beans, cooked	1 cup	4.6	17%
Black eyed peas, cooked	1 cup	4.3	16%
Sesame seeds	1 Oz	4.1	15%
Lima beans, cooked	1 cup	4	15%
Swiss chard, cooked	1 cup	4	15%
Oats, cooked	½ cup	3.7	14%
Kidney beans, cooked	1 cup	3.3	12%
Chickpeas, cooked	1 cup	3.2	12%
Beef chuck braised	3 oz	2.7	10%
Collard greens, cooked	1 cup	2.2	8%
Eggs, cooked	2 large	1.8	7%
Almonds	1 oz	1.3	5%

* Based on RDA for pregnant women (27mg/day).
Note: Bioavailability of iron in plant foods, in particular green leafy vegetables, is lower (USDA)
Source: Turner, 2019.

The absorption of heme iron is more uncontrolled than the absorption of non-heme iron. Should your body iron stores be well-repleted, non-heme iron is excreted from the body mostly through the stool, but the heme iron is readily absorbed and adds to iron stores, although they might be full. The problem with the generous absorption of heme iron is that it is a powerful source of free radicals, which have damaging effects to the body if not neutralized by anti-oxidants (Chavarro et al., 2008). What can be concluded from this information is that although heme iron is more bio-available than non-heme iron, this benefit is levelled by the oxidative stress that the body endures through absorption and over-storage of heme iron from animal sources. Good plant sources of non-heme iron include beans and legumes, and green, leafy vegetables, nuts, eggs, and whole grains (Chavarro et al., 2008). Good sources of non-heme iron are depicted in Table 8 above.

6.4.3.2. Bioavailability of Non-Heme Sources of Iron

Although iron from non-heme sources are more difficult to absorb than from heme sources, the absorption can be significantly improved by eating a high source of Vitamin C at the same meal, such as a fresh fruit salad, or other vegetables high in Vitamin C such as cauliflower, broccoli and other green leafy vegetables, especially those from the cruciferous (cabbage family) vegetables. Caffeine and tannins from tea and coffee suppress the absorption from non-heme iron from the gut in all people, and these drinks, if desired, should be taken at least 90 minutes or longer after a meal, so as not to interfere with the absorption of iron, especially in pregnancy. Pregnant women have an automatic increased absorption for non-heme iron, but a good iron supplement (preferably one which has at least 500mg of Vitamin C as part of the capsule) should be part of the supplemental protocol for pregnant women, and especially those who are vegan (Turner, 2019).

6.4.3.3. Benefits of Higher Protein

In contrast, some evidence suggests that a higher ratio of protein to carbohydrate for weight loss regimes holds some metabolic benefit. There is sound evidence that the higher satiety derived from a higher intake of protein assists in weight loss over time, and leads to a lower GL, due to reduction in carbohydrate intake (Noakes et al., 2005; Norman et al., 2002). Traditionally, diets that are high in carbohydrate and low in fat have been used to bring about weight loss and to improve metabolic and reproductive function, but there has been increased interest in the use of low carbohydrate/high protein diets (Moran et al., 2003). In comparison to both fat and carbohydrate, protein may assist in weight loss, due to its superior satiating power, and may improve lean body mass due to fat loss, with improved insulin sensitivity (Farshchi et al., 2007; Moran et al., 2003; Noakes et al., 2005; Norman et al., 2002).

Postprandial thermogenesis is also increased by protein intake, which could have favourable effects on abdominal fat (Farshchi et al., 2007). In 2005, a higher protein intake regime from lean red meat and dairy sources, restricted in energy, showed a weight loss advantage in patients suffering with elevated triglycerides, which is considered a strong marker for the presence of MS. The researchers found that subjects who consumed 30% protein from an energy-restricted diet reported experiencing less hunger than did those on a high-carbohydrate regimen. In addition, there were no detrimental effects on bone or renal metabolism of the higher protein regime over 12 weeks, and no difference between dietary composition (high protein as opposed to high carbohydrate, both with energy restriction) with regards to LDL cholesterol, HDL cholesterol, and glucose concentrations (Noakes et al., 2005). Studies elsewhere have also shown that low-fat, energy-restricted diets with higher protein content have a greater reducing effect on triglycerides, although weight loss was reported as being equal to that of the standard protein diet with caloric restriction (Marsh & Brand-Miller, 2005).

6.4.4. Fructose Excess and AGEs

The contributory mechanisms of both fructose and the non-enzymatical formation of AGEs to increased inflammation, development of MS, and in the case of fructose, the effect on appetite regulation, have been discussed elsewhere in this book. For decades, the glycative potential of different monosaccharides has been researched. Hyperglycemia is known for its potential to induce high rates of protein glycation, which can cause long-term metabolic complications. In 1981, researchers Bunn and Higgins were the first to publish a comparison among sugars for their non-enzymatic reactivity with haemoglobin, showing that fructose has a 7.5-fold higher reaction rate than glucose. A few years later, using bovine serum, it was showed that fructose had a glycoxidation rate of 10 times that of glucose (Aragno & Mastrocola, 2017).

The monosaccharides, glucose and fructose, largely exist as a stable ring structure in solution. Since only the open-chain form of a monosaccharide can react with an amino group of a protein to form a Schiff base, the higher reactivity of fructose is indicative of its higher quote of existing as an open chain in solution than glucose. Although the main glycating sugar in the human body is glucose, fructose can be produced under conditions of hyperglycemia through the polyol pathway, via sorbitol. This conversion process to fructose leads to the accumulation of fructose in the tissues, increasing the rate of AGE formation (Aragno & Mastrocola, 2017).

In the light of the observation that fructose is more reactive than glucose in generating glycation precursors, the modern consumption of high amounts of fructose, as compared to decades ago, is an important factor contributing to AGE formation. Among sugars most often used for sweetening in drinks and sweetened foods, fructose might represent the most hazardous for AGE accumulation. In individuals with NAFLD, population studies have found that the concomitant presence of MS is related to high fructose intake through sweetened beverages and foods. High fructose intake is strongly associated with elevated triglycerides and insulin resistance, paralleled by oxidative stress (Aragano & Mastrocola, 2017).

6.4.5. Dairy Products

The main sugar in milk, a di-saccharide, lactose, is digested in the gut to the single sugars, glucose and galactose. A condition known as premature ovarian failure (POF) often develops as a result of galactosemia, an inborn error of metabolism in which women cannot metabolize galactose. In animal studies, high intake of galactose has also been shown to lead to ovarian failure, and it were probably these notions that led to the hypothesis that high milk intake and dairy products may increase the risk of ovulatory infertility in healthy women, as published in 1994 by researchers Cramer et al. (Chavarro et al., 2007a). After their research study, very few human studies on this issue have been published, and the results have been inconsistent.

There is reason to believe that the intake of dairy products may be beneficial to ovarian function, and that different dairy products vary in their relation to fertility. In early 2000, studies showed that dairy intake may be associated with improved ovarian function. Low-fat dairy foods, but not full-fat dairy foods, have been associated with androgen excess, a prominent component of PCOS. Chavarro et al. (2007a) used a co-hort of healthy women from the NHS II, including more than 18 555 female nurses, to evaluate whether the intakes of low- and full- or high-fat dairy products, lactose and other nutrients concentrated in dairy foods were associated with anovulatory infertility. They found that in this study group, the intake of low-fat dairy foods was associated with a higher risk of anovulatory infertility, in contrast to the intake of full-fat or high-fat dairy, which seemed associated with a lower risk of anovulatory infertility. Moreover, there was no evidence that lactose intake was associated with anovulatory infertility, even though there was a wide range of intake of dairy products in the study population. No other associations were found between constituents of milk and other dairy products to anovulatory infertility, except for the inverse association between the fat content of dairy products and ovulatory infertility (Chavarro et al., 2007a).

The depth and detail of the NHS database allowed researchers Chavarro et al. (2008) to see clearly the foods that had the greatest effect on fertility. The most potent fertility food from the dairy group by far, was whole milk, ice cream. Low-fat products, such as low-fat yoghurt and sorbet, contributed most to ovulatory infertility.

Whole milk straight from the cow contains 4% per volume butterfat, varying according to the type of cow, and whether she was pregnant at the time of milking. However, all milk undergoes some fat-separation initially, leaving the full-fat milk products sold to the general product at a standardized 3.25% butterfat. The separation process then continues to generate two percent (2%) milk, and skim milk (containing less than 0.5% butterfat). Milk contains carbohydrates in the form of lactose, proteins in the form of casein and whey, butterfat, and water. The hormones and nutrients contained in milk could be either water- or fat-soluble.

6.4.5.1. Hormones in Milk

The hormones in milk affect human fertility more than any other component of dairy foods. Dairy products contain female hormones, such as prolactin, GnRH, estrogens and progesterone. It also contains a host of male hormones, such as testosterone and androstenedione, or their precursors. Female hormones, such as estrogen, would predominate naturally, since cows are females, and are milked for about 300 days per year, being pregnant much of this time (Chavarro et al., 2008, 113). Lastly, there are neutral hormones such as IGF-1.

The sex-hormones are mostly lipophilic (fat-preferring) and are found attached to fat globules in milk. The skimming or separation process removes much of the fat globules together with the hormones attached, leaving androgens, prolactin and IGF-1 behind in the watery part of the milk. This shift provides disbenefit to ovulation in the following ways:

- When male hormones are in excess of female hormones, unchecked, the maturation of follicles may be prevented.
- The presence of IGF-1 further exacerbates this by suppressing the production of SHBG by the liver. Having more affinity for testosterone than estrogen, a reduction of SHBG leaves a higher serum-testosterone to estrogen ratio.
- Excess prolactin, the hormone that stimulates milk production, may directly suppress ovulation, a dynamic which is well known, and the reason why lactating mothers do not fall pregnant easily.

The high potential of skim dairy products to cause elevated androgen levels was tested in the "Growing Up Today Study", involving more than 16 000 children of females enrolled in the NHS. Acne was significantly more prevalent in boys and girls who drank more skim-milk and low-fat yoghurt, than in those who consumed full-fat milk and full-fat yoghurt products. Interestingly, the study also looked at the "fatty foods" generally suspected to cause acne, such as pizza and chocolate consumption, and found no relation. The authors concluded that if milk influences the balance of sex hormones to the point of abundant serum-androgens for stimulating the sebaceous glands in the skin to cause acne, they could certainly affect the ovaries and other functional tissues in the human body (Chavarro et al., 2008).

6.4.5.2. Other Additions to Milk

When fat is removed from the milk, palatability aspects such as the creamy taste as well as the slightly yellow colour is lost. To compensate for these undesirable changes, milk producers add in small amounts of whey protein, of which alpha-lactalbumin is the most abundant. This milk protein, added to the diets of animals, respond with classic effects of male hormones, such as gain in lean muscle, and more efficient at exercise and training. Although there are no studies to back up that this is a fact, it is thought that the addition of alpha lactalbumin might have androgenic effects in the human body (Chavarro et al., 2007a).

6.4.5.3. Recommendations

In the absence of formal recommendations for milk and dairy intake in PCOS, it may be advisable for women, especially those suffering from acne, to limit the total intake of milk to two cups or less of full-fat milk per day, and pay attention to intake of other sources of calcium-rich foods, such as broccoli, kale, fish, and non-dairy milks, such as almond, hemp, rice, and coconut. Although milk is an excellent source of calcium, three cups of full cream milk is necessary to fulfil the daily requirement of 1 000 mg calcium in women. This comes with a high calorie and saturated fat content, which, in a PCOS woman trying to lose weight, might increase her already difficult task (Chavarro et al., 2008, Grassi, 2013).

6.4.6. Gluten

An internet search of gluten and PCOS will deliver tens, if not hundreds of diets and websites advocating the exclusion of gluten from a diet designed for PCOS. To date, no evidence-based information confirming the efficacy of gluten omission from the PCOS diet is available, to support this action (Grassi, 2013).

The true form of gluten allergy is a serious condition, celiac disease, which is an auto-immune intestinal disorder that affects no more than 1% of the general US population. Untreated, celiac disease has serious health consequences, such as intestinal damage, nutrient deficiencies, lethargy, irregular periods and infertility. Although the number of people diagnosed with celiac disease is not increasing, there has been a steady increase in the number of people, without the disease, trying to avoid gluten. This might be due to the belief that omitting gluten might lead to weight loss or increased energy (Grassi & Shur, 2019).

Non-celiac gluten sensitivity or intolerance has been described in roughly six times more cases than Americans who have celiac disease. The symptoms are often vague and range from fatigue, joint pain, bloating, gas, diarrhea and brain fog. Since gluten sensitivity does not cause intestinal damage, there are no associated nutritional deficiencies (Grassi & Shur, 2019).

Gluten is a mixture of two proteins in cereal products, which supplies the rigidity to baked goods and breads. It is found in wheat, rye, barley, oats, and products, such as beer, which are produced from these cereals. Gluten-containing cereals might easily be substituted by whole food starches and flours, such as potato, rice, and pea. With regards to the omission of all processed foods from the PCOS diet (as has been described before with regards to trans fat, AGEs, fructose-containing foods and additions to foods to compensate for the loss of extracted fat or other nutrients), the use of gluten-free products will return several highly-processed products into the diet. These gluten-free products often have higher caloric values and sugar contents, than the gluten-containing non-processed counterparts, making them poor food choices, especially for those with PCOS. Removal of gluten from a product also results in losses of other vitamins and fiber. A dietary specialist or registered dietician should evaluate and screen for symptoms of gluten sensitivity, and if necessary, have tests performed to establish the presence of celiac disease. There is no test to determine gluten sensitivity, so the recommendation would be to eliminate gluten and re-assess the problematic symptoms after a week (Grassi & Shur, 2019).

6.4.7. Food Cravings

Elevated levels of insulin are probably the cause of food cravings, especially for carbohydrate-rich foods that release glucose quickly such as sweets, chocolate, and other high-GI products. Having cravings is a frequently-reported symptom from females with PCOS, and although the craved food is not always sweets and chocolates, it might be savoury carbohydrates, such as deep-fried chips, pizza, and bread. Douglas et al. (2006) found that the dietary composition of PCOS women in comparison to non-PCOS women of the same BMI, race, and age group was similar in energy and macronutrient composition, but women with PCOS had a larger intake of high-GI foods. Their conclusion was that PCOS women probably do not eat that much more than non-PCOS women, but that the difference was in the type of food eaten. Furthermore, in the case of PCOS women, the food-intake constituted a higher intake of refined carbohydrates, possibly due to high levels of circulating insulin (Douglas et al., 2006: Grassi, 2013).

6.4.8. Meal Frequency and Snacking

The frequency of meals has lately been in the spotlight as an important aspect of human nutrition, profoundly affecting health and longevity (lifespan). Excessive energy intake is undoubtedly associated with chronic diseases, such as diabetes, and is a leading cause of death in the Western world. A hypo-energetic diet is important for prevention of chronic disease, and until now, the general notion has been to consume this intake divided into five or six smaller meals, *presuming* that this way of eating would reduce hunger and enhance reduction of body weight. Although evidence has been reported that reduced meal frequency could affect longevity, the effects of meal frequency on human health, remain somewhat unclear (Kahleova et al., 2014).

In animal studies, reduced meal frequency has shown to prevent the development of chronic diseases and extend the lifespan, due to lower oxidative damage, and improved stress tolerance/resistance. When mice were put under time-restricted feeding, eating the same number of calories from a high-fat diet as mice that were allowed ad-libitum feeding, they seemed to be protected from obesity, hyperinsulinemia and fatty infiltration of the liver (NASH). Intermittent fasting facilitates a prolonged lifespan and positively affects glucose tolerance, insulin sensitivity and the incidence of type-2 diabetes mellitus in mice. Emerging evidence also demonstrates a relationship between time-restricted feeding and weight regulation in animals (Kahleova et al., 2014).

Observational trials in humans have shown that eating more than three times daily may facilitate the development of overweight and obesity, and that frequent eating leads to a higher energy intake, by increasing food stimuli, making it difficult to control energy balance.

A randomized controlled trial in 2012, referred to by Kahleova et al, 2014, showed that more frequent eating showed no relation to reduced energy intake or body weight. It has also been demonstrated in type-2 diabetics that there might be more benefit for glycemic control to eat one larger meal, instead of two smaller meals, provided that the diet contained sufficient amounts of fiber. Larger, isocaloric mixed meals have also shown to cause a greater post-prandial thermogenic response, than should the same meal have been divided into six smaller meals. Observational data from humans has also suggested that the later in the day meals are eaten, the less success is achieved on weight loss therapy. It has been shown that fat storage is the greatest after the evening meal, and that eating breakfast may protect against weight gain in this regard (Kahleova et al., 2014).

Kahleova et al. (2014) performed a 24-week randomised crossover study, with the aim to examine the effect of meal frequency on body weight, liver fat infiltration, insulin resistance, and β-cell function, in type-2 diabetics. They compared the effect of six versus two (breakfast and lunch) meals, with the same caloric content, with each regimen lasting 12 weeks.

The study demonstrated a superior effect of the two-meal regime over the six-meal regime, with regards to body weight, liver fat infiltration, fasting glucose and insulin resistance. They further reported that the data from this study is consistent with that found in animal studies, which have shown the glucose-lowering effects of intermittent fasting regimes, such as fasting every other day, or fasting twice per week. This also improves glucose tolerance due to improved insulin sensitivity.

The data of the study by Kahleova et al. (2014) also contradicts the long-held belief that eating more frequently is "healthier" than eating less frequent, larger meals. Large, reliable studies have suggested that people who snack regularly are more prone to obesity and type-2 diabetes mellitus.

Periods of fasting between meals, may be of greater value to general health, than the actual composition of the diet. In one study, a high-fat diet, eaten in time-restricted meals, increased insulin sensitivity and decreased body weight, despite the high caloric content. As mentioned, there is evidence that eating meals later in the day, may disrupt success with weight loss, which cannot be explained through caloric difference, or energy expenditure. A potential explanation is that the timing of food intake can influence the circadian system, which must continuously adapt to and synchronize our physiological processes with the environment. Importantly, the circadian control of hunger and appetite had recently been demonstrated, and although the mechanisms for linking the timing of meals and maintenance of body weight are unknown, the satiety hormone, leptin, and the hunger hormone, ghrelin, might be involved. Changes in the levels of these hormones due to misalignment in circadian rhythm might very well influence energy intake and expenditure. A high-carbohydrate and high-protein breakfast my help prevent weight regain after weight loss, by reducing diet-induced compensatory changes in hunger, cravings, and especially ghrelin suppression (Kahleova et al., 2014).

Although further research is needed into the benefits of meal timing, Kahleova and colleagues (2014) concluded that two meals per day compared to an isocaloric six smaller meals per day-regime is superior in reduction of body weight, glucose tolerance, insulin sensitivity, and β-cell function.

Chapter 7

NEW DIETARY STRATEGIES FOR TREATMENT IN PCOS

7.1. INTRODUCTION

It is well known and cited throughout this book, that to date there are no known curative therapies for PCOS. Anti-diabetic and insulin-lowering medications might improve the insulin resistance and other metabolic abnormalities. However, given the strong connection of obesity and insulin resistance with PCOS, weight loss is recommended as the first line of treatment for women with PCOS. Moran et al. (2013) defined weight management as prevention of excess weight gain, and maintaining reduced weight in those subjects who are already overweight.

Dietary prescription for weight loss was, until recently thought to be one comprised of 50% of total calories as carbohydrate, 30% of total calories as fat, and 20% as protein. From the total caloric calculation per day, a minimum of 500 calories would have been subtracted, keeping the macronutrient distribution intact, and thought to make the weight loss difference. Despite this guideline, the specific dietary prescription to bring about the wanted weight loss together with metabolic and reproductive improvements, has been elusive (Marsh & Brand-Miller, 2005; Moran et al., 2013).

In the Thessaloniki Workshop Group (2008), the consensus group were already debating an "Atkins-type" diet, with very low calories. They reported that body weight in PCOS can be decreased in this manner by 12% over a time span of 24 weeks. Although different diets have been used to show that effective weight loss improved reproductive function, these studies failed to show that dietary patterns differentially affect weight loss and reproductive outcome, and the dropout rate continued to be high. The workshop concluded that diets with a reduced glycemic load (amount of carbohydrate) may be beneficial in stabilizing insulin sensitivity and reproductive health. The bottom line was that, whichever diet these women tried to follow, caloric intake should be cut by 500 calories per day, and weight loss of at least 5% from the original weight shown, before further medical interventions were to take place (Thessaloniki Workshop Group, 2008).

Despite the recommendations that lifestyle and dietary intake should be frontline to women with PCOS, the literature regarding dietary composition is sorely lacking. Not only does this pose considerable challenges to the researchers of PCOS and the optimal diet, but the entire picture of how to improve reproductive, metabolic, anthropometric, and physiological outcomes in these women remain blurred (Moran et al., 2013). Bearing this in mind, there is little value of going into each of the different diets assessed, as their negatives outweighed the positives, and might cause further confusion in the mind of the person reading this book.

7.2. What Do We Know for Sure?

We know that not only is caloric restriction important, but there are *many isolated areas in nutrition* that are scantly exposed or talked about, which could make a huge difference in overall reproductive function: Avoid trans fats completely; avoid AGEs; research lists of food further on the internet if you must; avoid fructose over-concentration by all accounts, and do not snack. If you are already taking an insulin-sensitizer, you should continue doing so, for as long as your infertility specialist deems it unnecessary.

The biggest secret for PCOS reproductive function restoration, is to *accept that females have a FINITE amount of days in which their egg cells or oocytes develop.* This starts 85 days in advance of a successful ovulation. Ovulation induction by means of drugs should therefore only start 3 to 4 months after dietary changes have been made and sustained. Be utterly and faithfully consistent to avoiding the single food-related issues that thwart fertility in those susceptible. It will be of no avail to quickly diet a week before you see your doctor or dietician to show some weight loss – it is the consistency that will have the greatest benefit to your reproductive cycle. Other pointers that we have learnt so far include:

- Eat one meal per day where you make vegetable protein the dominant protein.
- Stay as far away from trans fats as you possibly can.
- Avoid AGEs as far as possible.
- Avoid junk food. Nothing from a wrapper or a can or a plastic bag – ALL food should be whole, wholesome, fresh, excellent quality and cooked from scratch or eaten raw in the case of an already-edible form, such as nuts, avocado.
- Do not consume skim dairy products.
- DO NOT drink sugared drinks. This is one of the greatest interferences with your ovulation, other than trans fat. Do not even consider fruit juice or a sugar or fructose sweetened drink as a treat. Although our knowledge about artificial sweeteners is still severely lacking, the best advice would be to avoid them altogether, at least until your baby has been conceived and born.
- Take a multivitamin supplement that will give you at least 40 to 80 mg iron, and 400 mcg folic acid.
- Avoid pesticides and stay away from fields which are being sprayed.
- Do at least 30 minutes of moderate exercise per day, but do not overexert yourself with boot-camp or marathon running. Brisk walking, cycling or swimming a few laps go a long way to provide

you with the activity you need to help normalise your hormonal profile.

In the past 5 years or so, dietary strategies have surfaced and become very popular with the public, especially on social media. Furthermore, there are many motivational examples available, which make these strategies lucrative. The reader should bear in mind that whatever dietary regime they are prescribed, a well-informed professional dietician with all-round knowledge of the latest trends, would be the best option for help in this situation.

7.3. THE KETOGENIC AND LOW CARBOHYDRATE DIET

The ketogenic diet is one in which the carbohydrate content is reduced in favour of an increased fat, to a carbohydrate: fat ratio of 1:5. This diet was introduced in 1920. Therefore, the notion that fat can be eaten ad libitum and still induce weight loss, is not a recent one. Ketosis is the condition that follows when the body adapts from using mainly carbohydrate as fuel, to using mainly fat, both from the diet and from fat stores. Fatty acids, unlike glucose, are broken down into 2-carbon particles known as ketone bodies, which have the capacity to fuel the body and brain, the two most prominent ketones being β-hydroxybuturate and acetoacetate. Throughout human existence, mild ketosis has been a natural phenomenon in humans during fasting and lactation. Additionally, ketosis has a significant effect on suppressing hunger. Thus, a ketogenic diet is a good regulator of caloric intake, and mimics the effects of starvation, with regards to appetite control. A typical ketogenic diet for weight loss would consist of no more than 20g to 30g of carbohydrate in the form of mainly green vegetables and small amounts of other low GL vegetables and starch, 100g of protein in the form of full-fat dairy, meat, fish chicken, and eggs, and nuts, avocado pear and saturated fats, such as butter, mono-unsaturated fats, such as olive and avocado oils and polyunsaturated fats added to meals to enhance the fat content (Dasthi et al., 2004).

Current advances in medical nutrition have discounted the previous apprehensions about ketosis, and showed its benefits with regards to weight loss and metabolic restoration from obesity. It has been shown that generation of ketone bodies by the liver during fasting is essential to spare destruction of lean body mass for glucose synthesis. A ketogenic diet offers great value for weight reduction in obese patients, and has shown significant improvement in the levels of triglycerides, total cholesterol, LDL-cholesterol and glucose, and significant increases in HDL-cholesterol in patients. The side effects of drugs commonly used for weight loss and treatment of other metabolic disturbances were absent while following a ketogenic diet, indicating that following a ketogenic diet for a relatively long period of time is safe (Dasthi et al., 2004).

In 2005, Mavropoulos et al. published a pilot study of 11 women with PCOS, with a BMI of more than 27, on a ketogenic diet for 24 weeks. The subjects were put on a diet consisting of less than 20g of carbohydrate per day, ad libitum intake of full fat animal foods (meat, fish, chicken, eggs, milk and cheese) with 3 full cups of salad vegetables daily. The subjects were encouraged to drink 8 glasses of water per day and restrict their intake of alcohol and caffeine.

The study showed that the low-carbohydrate, ketogenic diet led to improvements in body weight, free testosterone, LH/FSH ratio, fasting serum insulin and symptoms associated with PCOS. The hyperinsulinemia of PCOS, which appears to increase androgen secretion from the ovaries, as well as the reduction in the production of SHBG, seemed to be reversed by the ketogenic diet. The researchers suggested that further studies should be conducted to ascertain whether the benefits were from the weight loss or from the actual carbohydrate restriction (Mavropoulos et al., 2005).

A study by Goss et al. (2014) was executed to determine whether, in women with PCOS, a diet moderately restricted in carbohydrate (41% carbohydrate, 19% protein, and 40% fat), would reduce total and regional adipose tissue during weight maintenance conditions, as compared to a eucaloric standard diet (55% carbohydrate, 18% protein, and 27% fat). The study was designed as a crossover intervention where subjects consumed a low-carbohydrate diet for 8 weeks, and a standard diet for 8 weeks, separated by a wash-out period of 4 weeks. All food was provided to the participants for each 8-week arm of the study, and were blinded to the diet order, either first consuming the low-carbohydrate diet of the standard diet for the first 8 weeks (Goss et al., 2014).

The results of the study showed a significant loss of both subcutaneous and intra-abdominal fat, as well as thigh-intra-muscular fat (an ectopic adipose tissue depot located between muscle groups and fibers, and associated with numerous diabetic and CVD risk factors) on the low-carbohydrate diet, in comparison to the standard diet, which led to a decrease in lean body mass. A similar, small amount of weight loss occurred in both arms of the study, and was unlikely to have influenced the results. The mechanisms underlying the greater loss of adipose tissue on the low-carbohydrate diet, independent of caloric restriction, may be related to insulin secretion. By lowering post-prandial insulin, adipogenesis is decreased, lipolysis is enhanced, promoting the use of adipose tissue as a fuel source, reducing adipocyte size, and limiting the development of new adipose tissue.

The authors concluded from this tightly-controlled crossover dietary intervention, that women with PCOS consuming a low-carbohydrate diet for maintenance of reduced body mass, resulted in profound improvements in body composition and fat distribution, while in contrast, following a high-carbohydrate diet resulted in loss of lean body mass in favour of increased fat mass (Goss et al., 2014).

7.4. Intermittent Fasting

Fasting is a millennia-old practice and discipline, both as a long-term and short-term restriction of food for both health and spiritual purposes. Light has been shed recently on the role that fasting may play in improving longevity, optimizing energy metabolism and increasing cellular protection. Intermittent fasting has the potential to delay ageing and help disease-prevention, while avoiding the side-effects caused by drug treatment (Weidemann & Brand, 2016).

Professor Tess van der Merwe, endocrinologist and honorary Professor at the University of Pretoria, wrote in the foreword of the work of Weidemann and Brand (2016) that hormesis, the scientific terminology for the adaptive response to mild stress, first entered the literature in 1943, from a publication by Southam and Erlich. Decades of refined research lapsed before the concept found a foothold in scientific literature, and in 2012 the number of citations exceeded 4 500.

Edward J. Calabrese, known as the father of modern day hormesis, lay the foundation for the science of hormesis. One field in which the principles of hormesis can be applied astutely is periodic or intermittent fasting, where the stress of caloric restriction can elicit the cytoprotective (cell-protection) effect to improve health, and more so in the diabetic and overweight population. Possible mechanisms by which fasting confers health benefits is an increase in mitochondrial metabolism, increased activity of the hypothalamic-pituitary-adrenal axis, and activation or SIRT-1 for cellular defense. The major health benefits are improvement in glucose metabolism, improved insulin sensitivity, cardio-protection, and diminished age-related diseases and brain deterioration.

7.4.1. Methods of Intermittent Fasting as a Lifestyle

Fasting can be done on alternative days, random days, or consecutive days. In 2013, Mosely and Spencer published a book with the title "The Fast Diet" which immediately became a bestseller, and describes the benefits of restricting energy severely for two days per week, while eating normally for five days per week. Although the internet overflows with intermittent fasting regimens for beginner-fasters and more long-term fasts, most of the observations and data from fasting studies are still derived from animal experimental studies (Patterson et al., 2016).

Two methods of energy restriction to favour weight loss have been examined: chronic caloric restriction (CR) and total calorie desistance (TCD) of fasting. Both methods of energy restriction improve metabolic health and other markers of health and longevity, such as reduced risk of atherosclerosis and improved insulin sensitivity. Studies on alternate-day fasting have shown that compliance with this regimen is greater and leads to less dropout, because the periodic nature of fasting mitigates the constant hunger that chronic CR subjects have to endure. Both CR and TCD need further research, but since the health benefits of TCD are at least as strong as CR, the less frequent but more intense energy deprivation of TCD might be preferred in the longer term (Horne, Muhlestein & Anderson, 2015).

The 5:2 method of intermittent fasting, also known as the 16/8 method, is the most practical experience according to Mosely and Spencer (2013) and Weidemann and Brand (2016). On the two fasting days per week, calories are limited to 600 per day, and divided into two meals, preferably breakfast and lunch. These two meals are eaten in the first 8-hour window of the day, and a 16-hour period of fasting follows, including the night sleep time, until the first meal of the next day.

Note from the author: After teaching and experiencing the results of intermittent fasting for more than eight years, it is clear that by doing a supper-skipping, rather than a breakfast-skipping fast to obtain 16 hours of fasting, the supper-skipping is more advantageous towards weight loss, and brings about results faster.

Intermittent fasting allows the high circulating levels of insulin to reduce to normal, and stimulates lipolysis, whereby the fat tissue of the body starts being used as fuel, inducing the state of ketosis. Intermittent or periodic fasting has been shown to have a beneficial effect on insulin sensitivity, compared with full-time dieters who lost the same amount of weight. Fasting for two to four consecutive days is an effective way to lose and maintain the lost weight, but the best results are seen with a regime which is practical and sustainable, depending on the individual (Weidemann & Brand, 2016).

Much research has been done by Dr Christa Varady, of the University of Chicago, Illinois. Varady (2011) reported that the same weight loss with alternate-day-fasting as with full-time dieting, but that fasting offered more benefits with regards to body composition. During fasting, human growth-hormone levels rise, which indicates preservation of muscle mass, to the detriment of fat mass.

7.4.2. Combining Ketogenesis with Intermittent Fasting

The internet and social media abound with testimonials from the effects of combining a ketogenic diet with periods of intermittent fasting. Very little information is available about the safety of this regime in women with PCOS wanting to fall pregnant, but the notion that the combination is highly effective for at least weight loss, cannot be ignored. From a medical and scientific point of view, this regime should be done to lose weight before trying to conceive, and with conception, a professional with extensive insight and knowledge into PCOS should be consulted for the way forward.

7.5. OVERCOMING THE "DIET" MENTALITY

We live in a society where indulgence is viewed as a virtue and discipline as punishment, which questions whether we believe in eating junk food, or whether we can help it. We have somehow come to the belief that there must be something we can eat or drink that can help us lose weight, and become slender and healthy. Although certain foods are better for our health than others, the idea that "more is better" has obstructed our view of moderation in everything that we eat and drink. (Weidemann & Brand, 2016).

Unfortunately, through brainwashing over the last 30 decades or so, people have come to believe that the only way to lose weight is through "dieting'. Although all diets have some restriction in common, they are all flawed in some way. Once a diet is stopped, the weight is very easily regained, plus some. The "diet mentality" often instils a self-destructive pattern of thought and behaviour. There are many reports of overindulgence before starting a diet, or craving of certain foods, merely because they are "forbidden". Most people regard dieting as a finite process, after which one might return to previous eating habits, after the wanted weight loss has occurred. With periodic fasting, the need for "rewards" or "treats" is reduced, and the improvement in general health brought about by intermittent fasting results in reduced cravings and desire for food-based rewards (Weidemann & Brand, 2016).

7.6. A Final Word

Although there are no known curative therapies for PCOS, anti-diabetic and insulin-lowering medications might improve the insulin resistance and other metabolic abnormalities. Weight loss is still recommended as the first line of treatment for women with PCOS, given the strong connection of obesity and insulin resistance with PCOS. However, optimal management of PCOS is achieved through a multi-disciplinary approach. Lifelong lifestyle management has been shown to improve the reproductive, metabolic and psychological aspects of PCOS best.

Life phases, such as pregnancy, lactation, and menopause might have a few different facets for the woman with PCOS than the non-PCOS woman, but in-depth discussion of this falls beyond the scope of this book. Since PCOS is a gender-specific metabolic syndrome, affecting all aspects of a woman's metabolic health, this is a condition that has no finite point at which the sufferer should stop caring about her health and take it for granted. Regular health check-ups should become an integral part of the life of the woman with PCOS. A healthy diet, based on good quality raw or cooked food should always form the basis of nutrition. Junk food and processed food has no place in the lifestyle and health care of women with PCOS.

REFERENCES

An, Y., Sun, Z., Zhang, Y., Liu, B., Guan, Y. and Lu, M. 2014. The use of berberine for women with polycystic ovary syndrome undergoing IVF treatment. *Clinical Endocrinology,* 80: 425-431. doi: 10.1111/cen.12294.

Agapova, S. E., Cameo, T., Sopher, A. B. and Oberfield, S. E. 2014. Diagnosis and Challenges of Polycystic Ovary Syndrome in Adolescence. *Seminars in Reproductive Medicine*, May, 32(3): 194-201. doi: 10.1055/s-0034-1371091.

Aragno, M. and Mastrocola, R. 2017. Dietary Sugars and Endogenous Formation of Advanced Glycation End products: Emerging Mechanisms of Disease. *Nutrients.* April, 9(4): 385. doi: 10.3390/nu9040385.

Arihara, K., Zhou, L. and Ohata, M. 2017. Chapter Five: Bioactive Properties of Maillard Reaction Products Generated from Food Protein-derived Peptides. *Advances in Food and Nutrition Research*, 81, 161-185. https://www.sciencedirect.com/science/article/pii/S1043452616300651.

Arora, M. 2017. *World Clinics Obstetrics and Gynaecology: Polycystic Ovary Syndrome.* July, 6(1). https://www.amazon.co.uk/World-Clinics-Obstetrics-Gynecology-Polycystic/dp/9352700694.

Azziz, R., Carmina, E., Dewailly, D., Diamanti-Kandarakis, E., Escobar-Morreale, H. F., Futterweit, W., Janssen, O. E., Legro, R. S., Norman,

R.J., Taylor, A.E. and Witchel, S.F. 2009. The Androgen Excess and PCOS Society criteria for the polycystic ovary syndrome: the complete task force report. *Fertility and Sterility*, February, 91(2): 456-488. Retrieved from Task Force on the Phenotype of the Polycystic Ovary Syndrome of The Androgen Excess and PCOS Society. https://www.fertstert.org/article/S0015-0282(08)01392-7/fulltext.

Azziz, R., Dumesic, D. A. and Goodarzi, M. O. 2011. Polycystic Ovary Syndrome: An Ancient Disorder? *Fertility and Sterility*, April, 95(5): 1544-1548. https://doi.org/10.1016/j.fertnstert.2010.09.032.

Barthelmess, E. K. and Naz, R. K. 2014. Polycystic ovary syndrome: Current status and future perspective. *Front Biosci (Elite Ed)*, January, 1(6): 104-119.

Basciano, H., Federico, L. and Adeli, K. 2005. Fructose, insulin resistance, and metabolic dyslipidemia. *Nutr Metab*, Feb, 21, 2(1): 5.

Bray, G. A., Nielsen, S. J. and Popkin, B. M. 2004. Consumption of high-fructose corn syrup in beverages may play a role in the epidemic of obesity. *American Journal of Clinical Nutrition*, 79: 537-543.

Broughton, D. E. and Moley, K. H. 2017. Obesity and female infertility: Potential mediators of obesity's impact. *Fertility and Sterility*, 107(4):840-847.

Chavarro, J. E., Rich-Edwards, J. W., Rosner, B. and Willett, W.C. 2007a. A prospective study of dairy foods intake and anovulatory infertility. *Human Reproduction*, 22(5): 1340-1347. doi: 10.1093/humanrep/dem 019.

Chavarro, J. E., Rich-Edwards, J. W., Rosner, B. A. and Willett, W. C. 2007b. Dietary fatty acid intakes and the risk of ovulatory infertility. *American Journal of Clinical Nutrition*, 85: 231-237.

Chavarro, J. E., Willett, W. C. and Skerrett, P. J. 2008. *The Fertility Diet*. New York, NY: McGraw Hill.

Dasthi, H. M., Mathew, T. C., Hussein, T., Asfar, S. K., Behbahani, A., Khoursheedn, M. A., Al-Sayer, H.M., Bo-Abbas, Y. Y. and Al-Zaid, N. S. 2004. Long-term effect of a ketogenic diet in obese patients. *Experimental and Clinical Cardiology*, 9(3): 200-205.

Dobe, M., Geisler, A., Hoffmann, D., Kleber, M., von Köding, P., Lass, N., Müther, S., Pohl, B., Rose, K., Schadfer, A., Többens, M.L., Vierhaus, R., Winkel, K. and Reinehr, T. 2011. The Obeldicks concept. An example for a successful outpatient lifestyle intervention for overweight or obese children and adolescents. *Bundesgesundheidsblatt Gesundheitsforschung Gesundheitsshutz,* May, 54(5): 628-635. doi: 10.1007/s 00103-011-1261-x.

Dokras, A., Stener-Victorin, E., Yildiz, B. O., Li, R., Ottey, S., Shah, D., Epperson, N. and Teede, H. Androgen Excess – Polycystic Ovary Syndrome Society: Position statement on depression, anxiety, quality of life, and eating disorders in polycystic ovary syndrome. 2018. *Fertility and Sterility.* May, 109(5). https://doi.org/10.1016/j.fertnstert.2018.01.038.

Douglas, C. C., Gower, B. A., Darnell, B. E., Ovalle, F., Oster, R. A. and Azziz, R. 2006. Role of diet in the treatment of polycystic ovary syndrome. *Fertility and Sterility,* March, 85(3): 679-688.

Elliott, S. S., Keim, N. L., Stern, K. S., Teff, K. and Havel, P.J. 2002. Fructose, weight gain, and the insulin resistance syndrome. *American Journal of Clinical Nutrition,* 76: 911-922.

Essah, P. A. and Nestler, J. E. 2006. The metabolic syndrome in polycystic ovary syndrome. *Journal of Endocrinological Investment*, 29(3), 270-280. doi: 10.1007/BF03345554.

Farshchi, H., Rane, A., Love, A. and Kennedy, R. L. 2007. Diet and nutrition in polycystic ovary syndrome (PCOS): Pointers for nutritional management. *Journal of Obstetrics and Gynecology,* Nov, 27(8): 762-773.

Field, C. J. 2006. Trans Fats: Beyond June 2006. *Canadian Council of Food and Nutrition.* https://www.cfdr.ca/Downloads/CCFN-docs/ Watching-Brief-on-TRANS-Fat---Feb25-_2_aspx.

Figueiredo, P. S., Inada, A. C., Fernandes, M. R., Arakaki, D. G., Freitas, K. de C., Guimaraes, R. de C. A., do Nascimento, V. A. and Hiane, P. A. 2018. An Overview of Novel Dietary Supplements and Food Ingredients in Patients with Metabolic Syndrome and Non-Alcoholic Fatty Liver

Disease. *Molecules*, 23(4): 877. https://doi.org/10.3390/molecules 23040877.

Funder, J. W., Krozowski, Z., Myles, K., Sato, A., Sheppard, K. E. and Young, M. 1997. Mineralocorticoid receptors, salt, and hypertension. *Recent Progress in Hormone Research*, 52: 247-260. PMID 9238855.

Gambineri, A., Patton, L., Altieri, P., Pagotto, U., Pizzi, C., Manzoli, L. and Pasquali, R. 2012. Polycystic Ovary Syndrome Is a Risk Factor for Type 2 Diabetes. *Diabetes,* Sept, 61: 2369-2371. doi: 10.2337/db11-1360.

Garg, D. and Merhi, Z. 2016. Relationship between Advanced Glycation End Products and Steroidogenesis in PCOS. *Reproductive Biology and Endocrinology,* 14: 71. doi: 10.1186/s12958-016-0205-6.

Gaskins, A. J. and Chavarro, J. E. 2018. Diet and Fertility: A review. *American Journal of Obstetrics and Gynecology,* April. https://dx.doi.org/10.1016/j-ajog.2017.08.010.

Gaskins, A. J., Mumford, S. L., Chavarro, J. E., Ahang, C., Pollack, A. Z., Wactawski-Wende, J., Perkins, N.J. and Sisterman, E.F. 2012. The Impact of Dietary Folate Intake on Reproductive Function in Premenopausal Women: A Prospective Cohort Study. *PLoS ONE,* September, 7(9): e46276. doi: 10.1371/journal.pone.0046276.

Gaysina, D. May 2, 2018. Folic acid in pregnancy – MTHFR gene explains why the benefits may differ. *The Conversation.* http://theconversation.com/folic-acid-in-pregnancy-mthfr-gene-esplains-why-the-benefits-may-differ-95302.

Gerhard, I., Monga, B., Waldbrenner, A. and Runnebaum, B. 1998. Heavy metals and fertility. *Journal of Toxicology and Environmental Health. Part A,* August, 54(8): 593-611.

Gilling-Smith, C., Story, H., Rogers, V. and Franks, S. 1997. Evidence for a primary abnormality of thecal cell steroidogenesis in the polycystic ovary syndrome. *Clinical Endocrinology,* 47: 93-99.

González, F. 2015. Nutrient-Induced Inflammation in Polycystic Ovary Syndrome: Role in the Development of Metabolic Aberration and Ovarian Dysfunction. *Semin Reprod Med*, 33: 276-286. http://dx.doi.org/10.1055/s-0035-1554918.

Goss, A. M., Chandler-Laney, P. C., Ovalle, F, Goree, L. L., Azziz, R., Desmond, R.A., Bates, G.W. and Gower, B.A. 2014. Effects of a eucaloric reduced-carbohydrate diet on body composition and fat distribution in women with PCOS. *Metabolism*, 63(10): 1257-1264. doi: 10.1016/j.metabol.2014.07.007.

Grassi, A. 2013. *PCOS: The Dietician's Guide.* Luca Publishing, Haverford PA 19041. ISBN: 978-0-9851164-2-5.

Grassi, A., and Shur, M. 2019. Is There a Connection Between Gluten and PCOS? *Very well Health,* January 2. https://www.verywellhealth.com/gluten-and-pcos-is-there-a-connection-2616491.

Guet, P., Royère, D., Paris, A., Lansac, J. and Driancourt, M. A. 1999. Aromatase activity of human granulosa cells in vitro: Effects of gonadotropins and follicular fluid. *Human Reproduction,* May, (1495): 1182-1189. https://doi.org/10.1093/humrep/14.5.1182.).

Gurevich, R. and Sadatay, A. 2018. How Ovarian and Antral Follicles Relate to Fertility: Understand what they are, what they do, and how many you should have. *Very well Family,* February 26. https://www.verywellfamily.com/follicle-female-reproductive-system-1960072?print.

Havel, P. J. 2005. Dietary fructose: Implications for dysregulation of energy homeostatis and lipid/carbohydrate metabolism. *Nutr Rev*, 63(5): 133-157.

Herriot, A. M., Whitcroft, S. and Jeanes, Y. 2008. A retrospective audit of patients with polycystic ovary syndrome: The effects of a reduced glycaemic load diet. *Journal of Human Nutrition and Dietetics*, August, 21(4), 337-345. doi: 10.1111/j.1365-277X2008.00890.x.

Horne, B. D., Muhlestein, J. B., and Anderson, J. L. 2015. Health effects of intermittent fasting: hormesis or harm? A systematic review. *American Journal of Clinical Nutrition*, 102: 464-470. https:// academic.oup.com/ajcn/article-abstract/102/2/464/4564588 on 20 October 2018.

Holt, S. H. A., Brand-Miller, A. C. and Petocz, P. 1997. An insulin index of foods: The insulin demand generated by 1000-kJ portions of common foods. *American Journal of Clinical Nutrition,* 66: 1264-1276.

Huang, P. L. 2009. A comprehensive definition for metabolic syndrome. *Disease Models and Mechanisms,* May, 2(5-6): 231-237. doi: 10.1242/dmm.001180.

Huber-Buchholz, M. M., Carey, D. G. P. and Norman, R. J. 1999. Restoration of reproductive potential by lifestyle modification in obese polycystic ovarian syndrome: Role of insulin sensitivity and luteinizing hormone. *J Clinical Endocrinol Metab,* 84(4): 1470-1474.

Jenkins, D. J. A., Wolever, T. M. S., Taylor, R. H., Barker, H., Fielden H. et al. 1981. Glycemic index of foods: A physiological basis for carbohydrate exchange. *American Journal of Clinical Nutrition,* 34: 362-366.

Kahleova, H., Belinova, L., Malinska, H., Oliyarnyk, O., Trnovska, J., Skop, V., Kazdova, L., Dezortova, M., Hajek, M., Tura, A., Hill, M. and Pelikanova, T. 2014. Eating two larger meals a day (breakfast and lunch) is more effective than six smaller meals in a reduced-energy regimen for patients with type-2 diabetes: A randomised crossover study. *Diabetologia,* 57: 1552-1560. doi: 10.1007/s00125-014-3253-5.

Kandaraki, E., Christakou, C. and Diamanti-Kandarakis, E. 2009. Metabolic syndrome and polycystic ovarian syndrome…and vice versa. *Arq Bras Endocrinol Metab,* 53(2): 227-237.

Kar, S. 2013. Anthropometric, clinical, and metabolic comparisons of the four Rotterdam PCOS phenotypes: A prospective study of PCOS women. *Journal of Human Reproductive Sciences,* 6(3): 194-200. doi: 10.4103/0974-1208.121422.

Katoaka, J., Tassone, E.C., Misso, M., Joham, A. E., Steiner-Victorin, E., Teede, H. and Moran, L. J. 2017. Weight Management Interventions in Women with and without PCOS: A Systematic Review. *Nutrients,* 9(996). doi: 10.3390/nu9090996.

Khazan, O. 2013. When Trans Fats Were Healthy. *The Atlantic: Health,* November. http://www.theatlantic.com/health/archive/2013/11/whentrans-fats-were-healthy/281274/.

Klein A. 2018. Cause of polycystic ovary syndrome discovered at last. *The Daily Newsletter: New Scientist University of Melbourne,* May 14. https://www.newscientist.com/article/2168705-cause-of-polycystic-ovary-syndrome-discovered-at-last/. *Nature Medicine.* doi: 10.1038/s41 591-018-0035-5.

Learning Radiology. 2018. *Polycystic Ovary Syndrome (PCOS). Stein-Leventhal Syndrome.* http://learningradiology.com/archives06/COW% 20190-Stein-Leventhal%20Ovaries/steinleventhalcorrect.htm.

Lê, K. A. and Tappy, L. 2006. Metabolic effects of fructose. *Curr Opin Clin Nutr Metabol Care*, 9: 469-475.

Li, L., Li, C., Pan, P., Chen, X., Wu, X., Ng, E. H. and Yang, D. 2015. A Single Arm Pilot Study of Effects of Berberine on the Menstrual Pattern, Ovulation Rate, Hormonal and Metabolic Profiles in Anovulatory Chinese Women with Polycystic Ovary Syndrome. *PLoS ONE,* 10(12): e0144072. doi: 10.1371/journal.pone.0144072.

Lim, A. J. R., Huang, Z., Chua, S. E., Kramer, M. S. and Yong, E. 2016. Sleep Duration, Exercise, Shift Work and Polycystic Ovarian Syndrome-Related Outcomes in a Healthy Population: A Cross-Sectional Study. *PLoS One*, 11(11): e0167048. doi: 10.1371/journal.pone.0167048.

Lucidi, R. S. 2018. Polycystic Ovarian Syndrome. *Medscape,* February 28. https://emedicine.medscape.com/article/256806-print.

Macut, D., Bjekić-Macut, J., Rahelić, D. and Dorknić, R. 2017. Insulin and the polycystic ovary syndrome. *Diabetes Research and Clinical Practice*, 130: 163-170. https://dx.doi.org/10.1016/j.diabres.2017.06.011.

Magoffin, D. A. 2005. Ovarian theca cell. *International Journal of Biochemistry and Cell Biology,* July, 37(7): 1344-1349. doi:10.1016/j.biocel.2005.01.016.

Malik, V. S., Schulze, M. B. and Hu, F. B. 2006. Intake of sugar-sweetened beverages and weight gain: A systematic review. *American Journal of Clinical Nutrition,* 84: 274-288.

Marsh, K. and Brand-Miller, J. 2005. The optimal diet for women with polycystic ovary syndrome? *British Journal of Nutrition*, 94(8), 154-165. doi: 10.1079/BJN20051475.

Mavropoulos, J. C., Yance, W. S., Hepburn, J. and Westman, E. C. 2005. The effects of a low-carbohydrate, ketogenic diet on the polycystic ovary syndrome: A pilot study. *Nutrition and Metabolism*, 2:35. doi: 10.1186/1743-7075-2-35. https://nutritionandmetabolism.com/content/2/1/35.

Mayo Clinic. 2018. Mayo Clinic Staff: *In Vitro Fertilization (IVF)*. https://www.mayoclinic.org/tests-procedures/in-vitro-fertilization/about/pac-20384716.

Merhi, Z. 2014. Advanced glycation end products and their relevance in female reproduction: Review Article. *Human Reproduction*, 29(1): 135-145. doi: 10.1093/humrep/det383.

Moeller, S. M., Fryhofer, S.A., Osbahr, A. J. and Rabinowitz, C. B. 2009. The effects of high fructose corn syrup: Review. *J Am Coll Nutr*, 28(6): 619-626.

Moran, L. J., Brinkworth, G., Noakes, M. and Norman, R.J. 2006. Symposium: Diet, nutrition and exercise in reproduction. Effects of lifestyle modification and polycystic ovarian syndrome. *Reprod Biomed Online*, March, 12(5): 569-578.

Moran, L. J., Ko, H., Misso, M., Marsh, K., Noakes, M., Talbot, M., Frearson, M., Thondan, M., Stepto, N. and Teede, H. J. 2013. Dietary Composition in the Treatment of Polycystic Ovary Syndrome: A Systematic Review to Inform Evidence-Based Guidelines. *Journal of the Academy of Nutrition and Dietetics*, 113(4): 520-545. doi:10.1016/j.jand.2012.11.018.

Moran, L. J., Noakes, M., Clifton, P. M., Tomlinson, L., Galletly, C. and Norman R. J. 2003. Dietary composition in restoring reproductive and metabolic physiology in overweight women with polycystic ovarian syndrome. *Journal of Clinical Endocrinology and Metabolism*, 88(2): 812-819.

Moran, L. J., Noakes, M, Clifton, P. M, Wittert, G. A., Le Roux, C. W., Ghatei, M. A., Bloom, S.R. and Norman, R.J. 2007. Postprandial ghrelin, cholecystokinin, peptide YY and appetite before and after weight loss in overweight women with and without polycystic ovarian syndrome. *Am J Clin Nutr*, 86: 1603-1610.

Moran, L. J., Noakes, M., Clifton., P. M., Wittert, G. A., Tomlinson, L., Galletly, C., Luscombe, N. D. and Norman, R. J. 2004. Ghrelin and

Measures of Satiety are altered in Polycystic Ovary Syndrome but not differentially affected by Diet Composition. *Journal of Clinical Endocrinology and Metabolism,* 89(7): 3337-3344. doi: 10.1210/jc. 2003-031583.

Moran, L. J. and Norman, R. J. 2004. Understanding and managing disturbances in insulin metabolism and body weight in women with polycystic ovarian syndrome. *Best Practice and Research. Clinical Obstetrics and Gynaecology,* 18(5), 719-736. doi: 10.1016/j.bpobgyn. 2004.05.003.

Moran, L. J., Pasquali, R., Teede, H. J., Hoeger, K. M. and Norman, R. J. 2009. Treatment of obesity in polycystic ovary syndrome: A position statement of the Androgen Excess and Polycystic Ovary Syndrome Society. *Fertility and Sterility,* December, 92(6): 1966-1982.

Morrison, J. A, Glueck, C. J. and Wang, P. 2008. Dietary trans fatty acid intake is associated with increased fetal loss. *Fertility and Sterility,* August, 90(2): 385-390.

Mozaffarian, D., Katan, M. B., Ascherio, A., Stampfer, M. J. and Willett, W. C. 2006. Trans Fatty Acids and Cardiovascular Disease. *New England Journal of Medicine,* 354, 1601-1613. https://pdfs.semanticscholar.org/ad95/cd9ca2ebfaef49f2bf9e9e2fcdadfa57bda6.pdf

Myers, M. G., Heymsfield, S. B., Haft, C., Kahn, B. B., Laughlin, M., Leibel, R. L., Tschöp, M. H. and Yanovski, J. A. 2012. Challenges and opportunities of defining Clinical Leptin Resistance. *Cellular Metabolism,* February, 15(2): 150-156. doi: 10.1016/j.cmet.2012.002.

National Institutes of Health (NIH). 2012. *Evidence-Based Methodology Workshop on Polycystic Ovary Syndrome: Executive Summary.* Washington, USA: National Institutes of Health. December 3 to 5. doi: https://prevention.nih.gov/sites/default/files/2018-06/FinalReport.pdf.

Noakes, M., Keogh, J. B., Foster, P. R. and Clifton, P. M. 2005. Effect of an energy-restricted, high-protein, low-fat diet relative to a conventional high-carbohydrate, low-fat diet on weight loss, body composition, nutritional status, and markers of cardiovascular health in obese women. *Am J Clin Nutr,* 81: 1298-1306.

Nomair, A. M, Aref, N. K., Rizwan, F., Ezzo, O. H. and Hassan N. 2014. Serum leptin level in obese women with polycystic ovary syndrome, and its relation to insulin resistance. *Asian Pacific Journal of Reproduction*, 3(4): 288-294. doi: 10.1016/S2305-0500(14)60014-5.

Nordio, M. and Proietti, E. 2012. The Combined therapy with myo-inositol and D-Chiro-inositol reduces the risk of metabolic disease in PCOS overweight patients compared to myo-inositol supplementation alone. *European Review for Medical and Pharmological Sciences,* 16: 575-581.

Norman, R. J., Davies, M. J., Lord, J. and Moran, L. J. 2002. The role of lifestyle modification in polycystic ovarian syndrome. *Trends Endocrinol Metab*, August, 13(6): 251-257.

Nurses' Health Study (NHS). 2018. *The Nurses' Health Study and the Nurses' Health Study II (NHS II).* http://www.nurseshealthstudy.org/about-nhs/history.

Orsino A., Van Eyk, N. and Hamilton, J. 2005. Clinical Features, investigations and management of adolescents with polycystic ovary syndrome. *Paediatrics and Child Health*, December, 10(10): 602-608.

Othman, R. 2010. *Feedback control mechanisms,* September 15. http://cikgurozaini.blogspot.com/2010/09/feedback-control-mechanisms.html.

Park, K. Y. and Yetley A. E. 1973. Intakes and food sources of fructose in the United States. *Am J Clin Nutr*, 58(5 Suppl): 737S-747S.

Pasquali, R. 2006. Obesity and androgens: facts and perspectives. Special Contribution. *Fertility and Sterility,* 85(5): 1319-1340.

Patterson, R. E., Laughlin, G. A., Sears, D. D., LaCroix, A. Z., Marinac, C., Gallo, L. C., Hartman, S. J., Natarajan, L., Senger, C. M., Martinez, M. E. and Villasenor, A. 2015. Intermittent Fasting and Human Metabolic Human Health. *Journal of the Academy of Nutrition and Dietetics*, 115(8): 1203-1212. doi:101016/j.jand.2015.02.018.

Penaforte, F. R., Japur, C. C., Diez-Garcia, R. W. and Chiarello, P. G. 2011. Upper trunk fat assessment and its relationship with metabolic and biochemical variables and body fat in polycystic ovarian syndrome. *Journal of Human Nutrition and Dietetics*, February, 24(1): 39-46.

Penaforte, F. & Japur, C. & Troncon, F. R. & De Arruda, I. L., Diez-Garcia, RW. and García, P. 2009. Metabolic and nutritional interfaces in polycystic ovary syndrome: Considerations regarding obesity and dietary macronutrients. *Revista Chilena de Nutrición* (Chile), September, 3(36). doi:10.4067/S0717-75182009000300010.

Pertynska-Marczewska, M., Diamanti-Kandarakis, E., Zhang, J. and Merhi, Z. 2015. Advanced glycation end products: A link between metabolic and endothelial dysfunction in polycystic ovary syndrome? *Metabolism,* November, 64(11), 1564-1573. http://dx.doi.org/10.1016/j.metabol.2015.08.010.

Peter-Ross, E., Janet, L., Roux, K. and Allers, E. 2015. Cellular and molecular psychiatry special interest group: Treatable Genomic Polymorphisms of 5,10 Methyltetrahydrofolate Reductase (MTHFR). *South African Society of Psychiatrists (SASOP).* September.

Peterson, M. K. and Zu, K. 2016. Trans Fats: Current Scientific Update. *Food Safety Magazine*, February/March. https://www.foodsafetymagazine.com/magazine-archive1/februarymarch-2016/trans-fats-current-scientific-update/

Reinehr, T., Kulle, A., Rothermel, J., Knop, C., Lass, N., Bosse, C. and Holterhus, P-M. 2017. Weight loss in obese girls with polycystic ovarian syndrome is associated with a decrease in Anti-Muellerian Hormone concentrations. *Clinical Endocrinology,* 87: 187-193. doi: 10.1111/cen.13358.

Rencber, S. F., Ozbek, S. K., Eraldemir, C., Sezer, Z., Kurn, T., Ceylan, S. and Guzel, E. 2018. Effect of resveratrol and metformin on ovarian reserve and ultrastructure in PCOS: An experimental study. *Journal of Ovarian Research,* 11:55. https://doi.org/10.1186/s13048-018-0427-7.

Robinson, A., Chan, S-P., Spacey, S., Anyaoku, V., Johnston, D. G. and Franks, S. 1992. Postprandial thermogenesis is reduced in polycystic ovary syndrome and is associated with increased insulin resistance. *Clinical Endocrinology,* 36: 537-543. https://doi.org/10.1111/j.1365-2265.1992.tb02262.x.

Roe, A.H. and Dokras, A. 2011. The diagnosis of polycystic ovary syndrome in adolescents. *Reviews in Obstetrics and Gynaecology*, Summer, 4(2), 45-51.

Rotterdam. 2003. The Rotterdam ESHRE/ASRM sponsored PCOS consensus group. Revised 2003 consensus on diagnostic criteria and long-term health risk related to polycystic ovary syndrome (PCOS). *Human Reproduction*, 2004, 19(1): 41-47. https://doi.org/10.1093/humrep/deh098.

Rowe, K. 2019. Folic Acid vs. Folate: Everything you need to know. *Brain Health*, April 13. https://www.brainmdhealth.com/blog/folic-acid-vs-folate-everything-you-need-to-know/.

Rutchik, J.S. 2014. Organic Solvents: Background, Pathophysiology, Epidemiology. *Medscape*, May. https://emedicine.medscape.com/article/1174981_overview.

Saha, L., Kaur, S. and Saha, P. K. 2012. Pharmacotherapy of the polycystic ovary syndrome – an update. *Fundamental and Clinical Pharmacology*, 26: 54-62.

Saha, L., Kaur, S. and Saha, P. K. 2013. N-acetyl cysteine in clomiphene citrate resistant polycystic ovary syndrome: A review of reported outcomes. *Journal of Pharmacology and Pharmacotherapeutics*, 493: 187-191. doi: 10.4103/0976-500X.114597.

Sakumoto, T., Tokunaga, Y., Tanaka, H., Nohara, M., Motegi, E., Shinkawa T., Nakaza, A. and Higashi, M. 2010. Insulin resistance/hyperinsulinemia and reproductive disorders in infertile women. *Reproductive Medicine and Biology*, Sept, 9(4): 185-190. doi: 10.1007/s12522-010-0062-5.

Saleem, F. and Rizvi, S.W. 2017. New Therapeutic Approaches in Obesity and Metabolic Syndrome Associated with Polycystic Ovary Syndrome. *Cureus*, 9(11): e1844. doi: 10.7759/cureus.1844.

Schöfl, C., Horn, R., Schill, T., Schlösser, H. W., Muller, M. J. and Brabant, G. 2002. Circulating ghrelin levels in patients with polycystic ovary syndrome. *Journal of Clinical Endocrinology and Metabolism*, 87(10): 4607-4610.

Sears, B. and Perry, M. 2015. The role of fatty acids in insulin resistance. *Lipids in Health and Disease*, 14: 121. https://doi.org/10.1186/s12944-015-0123-1.

Siebert, T. I., Kruger, T. F. and Lombard, C. 2009. Evaluating the equivalence of clomiphene citrate with and without Metformin in ovulation induction in PCOS patients. *Journal of Assisted Reproduction and Genetics,* 26(4): 165-171.

Sikaris, K.A. 2004. The clinical biochemistry of obesity. Review article. *Clinical Biochemist Reviews,* August, 25: 165-181. https://www.ncbi.nlm.nih.gov/pmc/articles/PMC1880830/pdf/cbr25_3p165.pdf.

Silber, S. J. 2018. How does your biological clock work? *The Infertility Center of St. Louis.* https://www.infertile.com/beating-biological/

Silvestris, E., De Pergola, G., Rosania, R. and Loverro, G. 2018. Obesity as a disruptor of the female fertility. *Reproductive Biology and Endocrinology*, 16(22). https://doi.org/10.1186/s12958-018-0336-z.

Southam C. M., and Erlich J. 1943. Effects of extract of western red-cedar heartwood on certain wood-decaying fungi in culture. *Phytopathology.* 33: 517-524.

Stanhope, K.L. and Havel, P.J. 2008. Fructose consumption: Potential mechanisms for its effects to increase visceral adiposity and induce dyslipidemia and insulin resistance. *Curr Opin Lipidol,* 19: 16-24.

Stepto, N. K., Cassar, S., Joham, A. E., Hutchinson, S. K., Harrison, C. L., Goldstein, R. F. and Reede, H. J. 2013. Women with polycystic ovary syndrome have intrinsic insulin resistance on euglycaemic-hyperinsulinaemic clamp. *Human Reproduction,* 28(3): 777-784. doi: 10.1093/humrep/des/463.

Szydlarska, D., Machaj, M. and Jakimiuk, A. 2017. History of discovery of polycystic ovary syndrome. *Advances in Clinical and Experimental Medicine,* 26(3): 555-558. doi: 10.17219/acem/61987.

Tanguturi, S. C. and Nagarakanti, S. 2018. Polycystic ovary syndrome and periodontal disease; Underlying links – a review. *Indian Journal of Endocrinology and Metabolism,* 22(2): 267-273. http://wwwijem.in/text.asp?2018/22/2/267/232378.

Tappy, L. and Lê, K. 2010. Metabolic Effects of Fructose and the Worldwide Increase in Obesity. *Physiological Reviews*, January, 90(1), 23-46. https://www.physiology.org/doi/full/10.1152/physrev.00019. 2009.

Tarrago-Trani, M. T., Phillips, K. M., Lemar, L. E. and Holden, J. M. 2006. New and existing oils and fats used in products with reduced trans-fatty acid content. *Journal of the American Dietetics Association,* June, 106(6): 867-880. doi: 10.1016/j.jada.2006.03.010.

Teede, H. J., Hutchinson, S. K. and Zoungas, S. 2018. The management of insulin resistance in polycystic ovary syndrome. *TRENDS in Endocrinology and Metabolism*, 18(7): 273-279. doi: 10.1016/j.tem.2007.08.001.

Teff, K. L., Elliott, S. S., Tschöp, M., Kieffer, T. J., Rader, D., Heiman, M., Townsend, R. R., Kein, N. L., D'Alessio, D. and Havel, P.J. 2004. Dietary fructose reduces circulating insulin and leptin, attenuates postprandial suppression of ghrelin, and increases triglycerides in women. *Journal of Clinical Endocrinology and Metabolism,* 89(6): 2963-2072.

Thessaloniki workshop group. 2008. Thessaloniki ESHRE/ASRM-Sponsored PCOS Consensus Workshop Group. Consensus on infertility treatment related to polycystic ovary syndrome. *Human Reproduction,* 23(3): 462-477.

Thomson, R. L., Buckley, J. D., Lim, S. S., Noakes, M., Clifton, P. M., Norman, R. J. and Brinkworth, G. D. 2010. Lifestyle management improves quality of life and depression in overweight and obese women with polycystic ovary syndrome. *Fertility and Sterility,* October, 94(5). doi:10.1016j/fertnstert.2009.11.001.

Trumbo, P., Schlicker, S., Yates, A. A. and Poos, M. 2002. Dietary reference intakes for energy, carbohydrate, fiber, fat, fatty acids, cholesterol, protein and amino acids. *Journal of the American Dietetic Association*, 102(11), 1621-1630. https://doi.org/10.1016/S0002-8223(02)90346-9.

Turner, H. A. 2019. *Web Exclusive: Iron in pregnancy: Maintaining adequate intake for mother and child.* https://www.todaysdietitian.com/news/exclusive0116.shtml.

Tyagi, S., Gupta, P., Saini, A.S., Kaushal, C. and Sharma, S. 2011. The peroxisome proliferator-activated receptor: A family of nuclear receptors role in various diseases. *Journal of Advanced Pharmaceutical and Technology Research,* Oct-Dec, 2(4): 236-240. doi: 10.4103/2231-4040.90879.

University of Washington. 2018. *Polycystic ovary syndrome.* https://courses.washington.edu/conj/bess/reproductive/pcos.htm.

Uribarri, J., Del Castillo, M. D., De la Maza, M. P., Filip, R., Gugliucci, A., Luevano-Contreras, C., Macias-Cervantes, M. H., Bastos, D. H. M., Medrano, A., Menini, T., Portero-Otin, M., Rojas, A., Sampaio, G. R., Wrobel., K., Wrobel., K. and Garay-Sevilla, M. E. 2015. Dietary Advanced Glycation End Products and Their Role in Health and Disease. *Advances in Nutrition,* 6: 461-473. doi: 10.3945/an.115.008433.

Uribarri, J., Woodruff, S., Goodman, S., Chai, W., Chen, X., Pyzik, R., Yong, A., Striker, G. E. and Vlassara, H. 2010. Advanced glycation end products in foods and a practical guide to their reduction in the diet. *J Am Diet Assoc,* 110: 911-916.

US Occupational Safety and Health Administration. 2016. US Department of Labor. *Hazard Classification Guidance for Manufacturers, Importers, and Employers.* https://www.osha.gov/Publications/OSHA3844.pdf.

Varady, K.A. 2011. Intermittent versus daily calorie restriction: Which diet regimen is more effective for weight loss? *Obesity Reviews,* 12(7): 593-601.

Vogt, P.F. and Gerulis, J.J. 2005. Amines, Aromatic. *Ullmann's Encyclopedia of Industrial Chemistry.* Weinheim: Wiley-VCH. doi:10.1002/14356007.a02_037.

Von Wartburg, L. 2007. What's a glucose clamp, anyway? *Diabetes Health,* November 6. https://www.diabeteshealth.com/whats-a-glucose-clamp-anyway/

Vos, M. B., Kimmons, J. E., Gillespie, C., Welsh, J. and Blanck, H. M. 2008. Dietary fructose consumption among US children and adults: The third national health and nutrition examination survey. *Medscape J Med*, 10(7): 160.

Wei, W., Zhao, H., Wang, A., Siu, M., Liang, K., Deng, H., Ma, Y., Zhang, Y., Zhang, H. and Guan, Y. 2012. A clinical study on the short-term effect of berberine in comparison to metformin on the metabolic characteristics of women with polycystic ovary syndrome. *European Journal of Endocrinology*, January, 166: 99-105. doi: 10.1530/EJE-1190616.

Weidemann, A. 2012. "*The role of fructose restriction in addition to dietary modifications for weight loss and lifestyle improvement, on fertility outcome and other markers of metabolic syndrome (MS), in obese women with polycystic ovarian syndrome (PCOS)*". Thesis presented in partial fulfilment of the requirements for the degree of Master of Nutrition in the Faculty of Medicine and Health Sciences at Stellenbosch University, Stellenbosch, South Africa.

Weidemann, A. and Brand, A. 2016. *Periodic Fasting: Lose weight, feel great, live longer*. Cape Town, South Africa: Struik Lifestyle.

Wikipedia. 2019. *Peptide hormone.* https://en.wikipedia.org/wiki/Peptide_ hormone.

Wilson, C. 2019. *Female reproductive hormones. Slide show.* https://slide player.com/slide/5756143/

Young, J. M. and McNeilly, A. S. 2010. Theca: the forgotten cell of the ovarian follicle. *Reproduction,* 140(4): 489-504. doi: 10.1530/REP-10-0094.

Zhang, J. J. and Merhi, Z. 2016. Could advanced glycation end-products explain the poor response to controlled ovarian hyperstimulation in obese women? *Journal of Endocrinology and Diabetes*, 3(2): 1-9. doi: https://dx.doi.org/10.15226/2374-6890/3/2/0146.

AUTHOR'S CONTACT INFORMATION

Annchen Weidemann
Private practicing Dietician at West Coast Private Hospital,
Vredenburg, West Coast, South Africa
Email: annwei1963@gmail.com

INDEX

A

advanced glycation end-products (AGEs), ix, xi, xvii, xx, 47, 48, 49, 50, 51, 52, 53, 116, 128, 129, 133, 138, 139, 162
alpha linolenic acid (ALA), xvii
American Society for Reproductive Medicine (ASRM), xvii, 23, 158, 160
Androgen excess (H), xviii, 24, 35, 147, 148, 149, 150, 151, 152, 153, 154, 155, 156, 158, 159, 160, 161, 162
Androgen Excess and PCOS (Society) (AE-PCOS), xvii, 23, 24, 105, 114, 148
anti-Müllerian hormone (AMH), xvii, 67, 68, 93, 96, 106
apolipoprotein B100 (ApoB), xvii, 65
arachidonic acid (AA), xvii, 44, 98
artificial insemination (AI), xvii, 85
assisted reproductive technology (ART), xvii, 52, 81, 85, 119

B

binge-eating disorder (BED), xvii, 21
bioelectrical impedance (BI), xvii, 38
body mass index (BMI), xvii, 20, 32, 36, 38, 39, 40, 51, 53, 74, 77, 78, 81, 84, 86, 91, 99, 104, 106, 112, 118, 119, 134, 141

C

caloric restriction (CR), xvii, 93, 128, 138, 142, 143
cardiovascular disease (CVD), xviii, 25, 26, 33, 35, 37, 39, 40, 52, 54, 55, 86, 105, 112, 120, 142
central nervous system (CNS), xvii, 66, 79
cholecystokinin (CCK), xvii, 75, 76, 154
clomiphene citrate (CC), xvii, 83, 84, 89, 91, 158, 159
co-enzyme A (CoA), xvii, 64, 65
computed tomography (CT), xvii, 38
conjugated linoleic acid (CLA), xvii, 56
controlled ovarian hyperstimulation (COH), xvii, 50, 52, 162
C-reactive protein (CRP), xvii, 37, 43, 45, 47

D

D-chiro-inositol (DCI), xviii, 88
de novo lipogenesis (DNL), xviii, 57, 63, 64
Dehydroepiandrosterone DHEA), xviii, 13
Dehydroepiandrosterone sulfate (DHEA-S), xviii, 13
deoxyribonucleic acid (DNA), xviii, 5, 94
dietary folate equivalent (DFE), xviii, 94, 95
docosahexanoic acid (DHA), xviii, 98, 99

E

Eicosapentanoic acid (EPA), xviii, 98, 99
Estradiol (E2), xviii, 12
Estriol (E3), xviii, 12
Estrone (E1), xviii, 12
European Society for Human Reproduction and Embryology (ESHRE), xviii, 22, 158, 160

F

follicle stimulating hormone (FSH), xviii, 7, 12, 13, 15, 31, 68, 73, 74, 83, 95, 141
free fatty acids (FFA), xviii, 38, 43

G

generally regarded as safe (GRAS), xviii, 99, 120
glucose transporter type-4 (GLUT4), xviii, 29, 58
glucose transporter type-5 (GLUT5), xviii, 58
glycemic index (GI), 112
glycemic load (GL), xviii, 112, 114, 116, 122, 127, 138, 140
gonadotropin-releasing hormone (GnRH), xviii, 12, 13, 30, 41, 131

H

haemoglobin A1c (HbA1c), xviii, 86
health-related quality of health (HRQoL), xix, 20, 21
high-density lipoprotein (cholesterol) (HDL), xviii, 25, 33, 34, 55, 65, 105, 128, 141
high-fructose corn syrup (HFCS), xviii, 59, 60, 61, 148
homeostatic model assessment of insulin resistance (HOMA-IR), xix, 28, 93
human immunodeficiency virus (HIV), xviii, 91
hypothalamic-pituitary-ovarian-axis (HPO-axis), xix, 13, 27, 30, 39, 41, 44, 69, 73, 78, 101, 103

I

impaired glucose tolerance (IGT), xix, 25, 26, 32, 82, 105
in vitro fertilization (IVF), xix, 36, 40, 85, 89, 90, 147, 154
inositolphosphoglycans (IPGs), xix, 88
insulin resistance (IR), xix, 18, 24, 25, 26, 27, 28, 29, 30, 32, 33, 35, 37, 38, 39, 40, 42, 43, 44, 45, 46, 49, 54, 57, 62, 64, 66, 69, 71, 73, 74, 75, 76, 77, 78, 82, 84, 88, 89, 90, 91, 93, 97, 98, 99, 103, 104, 105, 111, 114, 115, 116, 120, 121, 129, 135, 136, 137, 146, 148, 149, 156, 157, 159, 160
insulin-like growth factor 1 (IGF-1), xix, 32, 131
interleukin-1 beta (IL-1β), xix, 93
interleukin-6 (IL-6), xix, 37, 39, 45, 93

L

leptin receptor (LEPR), xix, 40, 78, 79
low-density lipoprotein (cholesterol) (LDL), xix, 25, 55, 65, 86, 89, 93, 128, 141
luteinizing hormone (LH), xix, 12, 13, 15, 31, 32, 35, 37, 40, 41, 68, 69, 73, 74, 83, 99, 106, 141, 152

M

metabolic syndrome (MS), ix, xi, xix, 24, 25, 32, 33, 34, 37, 41, 49, 57, 62, 65, 66, 69, 82, 89, 101, 104, 105, 128, 129, 146, 149, 152, 162
methylenetetrahydrofolate (MTHFR), 94, 157
Myo-inositol (MI), xix, 88

N

N-acetyl-cysteine (NAC), xix, 91, 92
National Academy of Sciences (of the USA) (NAS), xix, 55, 56
National Institute of Clinical Excellence (NICE), xix, 81
National Institutes of Health (of the USA) (NIH), xix, 22, 23, 24, 116, 117, 155
non-alcoholic fatty liver disease (NAFLD), xix, 26, 44, 93, 129
non-alcoholic steatohepatitis (NASH), xix, 33, 135
non-steroidal anti-inflammatory drugs (NSAID'a), xix
nuclear factor kappa-B (NF-κB), xix, 46
Nurses' Health Study (NHS), xix, 116, 117, 118, 120, 121, 124, 125, 130, 131, 156

O

oligo/anovulation (O), xix, 4, 22, 23, 24, 26, 34, 39, 52, 69, 102, 103, 147, 148, 149, 152, 156
oral contraceptive pills (OCPs), 82
oral glucose tolerance test (OGTT), 62, 105
ovarian hyperstimulation syndrome (OHSS), 85

P

peroxisome proliferator-activated receptors (PPARs), xix, 54
phosphofructokinase (PFK), xix, 57, 58, 64
polycystic ovarian morphology (P), xix, 24, 34, 148, 149, 150, 151, 152, 153, 154, 155, 156, 157, 158, 159, 160, 161
poly-unsaturated fatty acid (PUFA), xx, 98, 99
premature ovarian failure (POF), xix, 129

Q

quality of life (QoL), xx, 20, 102, 107, 149, 160

R

randomized controlled trial (RCT), xx, 112, 119, 135
reactive oxygen species (ROS), xx
resting energy expenditure (REE), xx, 5, 39
ribonucleic acid (RNA), xx, 94
Royal College of Obstetricians and Gynaecologists (RCOG), xx, 26

S

sex hormone-binding globulin (SHBG), xx, 32, 35, 71, 83, 99, 131, 141
silent information regulator-1 (SIRT-1), xx, 92, 93, 143
Society of Obstetricians and Gynecologists of Canada (SOGC), xx, 81
soluble RAGE (sRAGE), xx, 49
sterol receptor-binding protein (SREBP), xx, 64

T

the cell receptor for AGEs (RAGE), xi, xx, 49, 50, 52
total caloric deprivation (TCD), xx, 143
troglitazone (TZD), xx, 87
tumour necrosis factor alpha (TNF-α), xx, 37, 39, 43, 45, 46, 93

type-2 diabetes mellitus (T2DM), xx, 25, 26, 32, 33, 35, 44, 46, 49, 54, 62, 69, 82, 84, 105, 120, 135, 136

U

United States of America (USA), xix, xx, 55, 56, 59, 60, 155
US Food and Drug Administration (FDA), xviii, 99, 120

V

very-low-density lipoprotein (VLDL), xx, 63, 64, 65

W

waist-hip-ratio (WHR), xx, 38
waistline circumference (WC), xx, 33, 38

Related Nova Publications

ALLELIC FORMS OF THE FMR1 GENE: FRAGILE X SYNDROME, PRIMARY OVARIAN INSUFFICIENCY AND TREMOR ATAXIA SYNDROME AMONG OTHERS

EDITOR: Montserrat Milà

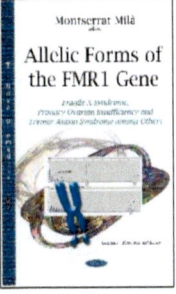

SERIES: Genetics – Research and Issues

BOOK DESCRIPTION: The FMR1 gene is an example of how a single gene can have different phenotypic effects. Indeed, since its discovery in 1991 it has revealed new facets: classic Fragile X syndrome (FXS), Fragile X premature ovarian insufficiency (FXPOI), Fragile X tremor-ataxia syndrome (FXTAS) and other emerging disorders from which we are continuously learning more about this gene.

HARDCOVER ISBN: 978-1-63321-914-4
RETAIL PRICE: $192

UTERINE FIBROIDS: EPIDEMIOLOGY, SYMPTOMS AND MANAGEMENT

EDITORS: Simone Ferrero, MD, PhD and Fabio Barra, MD

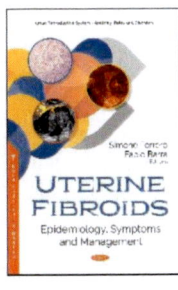

SERIES: Human Reproductive System – Anatomy, Roles and Disorders

BOOK DESCRIPTION: The aim of this book is to summarize the evidence regarding epidemiology, pathogenesis, clinical presentation, diagnosis and management of uterine myomas.

HARDCOVER ISBN: 978-1-53615-046-9
RETAIL PRICE: $195

To see a complete list of Nova publications, please visit our website at www.novapublishers.com

Related Nova Publications

CURSED? BIOLOGIC AND CULTURAL ASPECTS OF THE MENSTRUAL CYCLE AND MENSTRUATION

EDITOR: Elizabeth R. Bertone-Johnson

SERIES: Medicine and Biology Research Developments

BOOK DESCRIPTION: *Cursed? Biologic and Cultural Aspects of the Menstrual Cycle and Menstruation* explores in detail how menstruation and the menstrual cycle affect the lives of girls and women around the world. In addition to presenting current research on biologic and health issues surrounding menstruation and menstrual cycle function, authors discuss how menstruation directly impacts culture, art, feminism and gender politics, education and global development.

HARDCOVER ISBN: 978-1-53613-402-5
RETAIL PRICE: $160

AN ESSENTIAL GUIDE TO MEN'S AND WOMEN'S HEALTH

EDITORS: Allen Goodwin, Sheri Lynch

SERIES: Medicine and Biology Research Developments

BOOK DESCRIPTION: *An Essential Guide to Men's and Women's Health* provides a current summary of bone health in men. Topics include: the epidemiology and temporal trends of low bone mass, osteoporosis and related fractures; the morbidity and mortality associated with osteoporosis and osteoporotic fractures; low bone mass risk factors and etiology; and osteoporotic risk assessment.

SOFTCOVER ISBN: 978-1-53613-331-8
RETAIL PRICE: $95

To see a complete list of Nova publications, please visit our website at www.novapublishers.com